Z00006568

D1558496

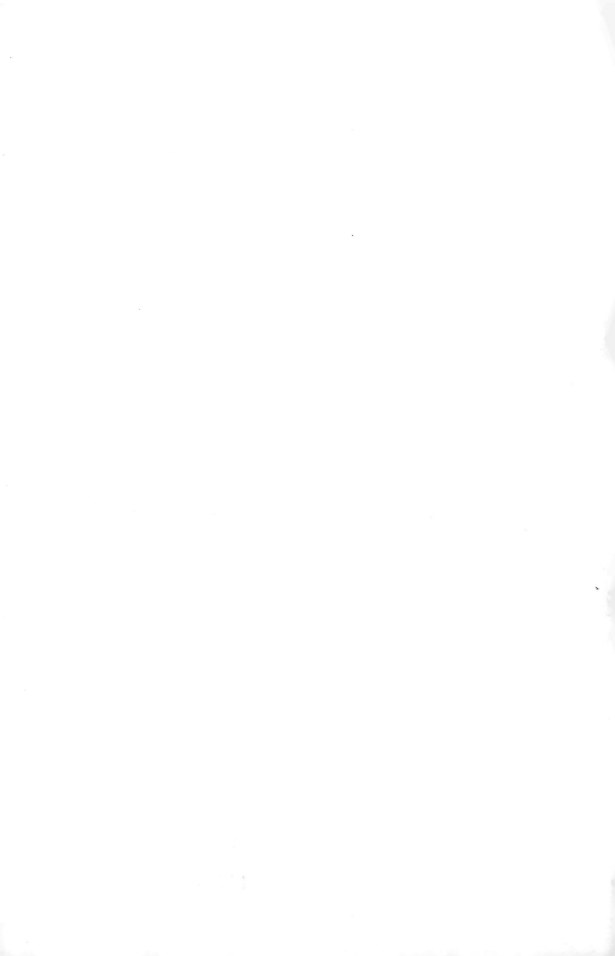

TRACHEOTOMY

Airway Management, Communication, and Swallowing

SECOND EDITION

TRACHEOTOMY

Airway Management, Communication, and Swallowing

SECOND EDITION

Eugene N. Myers, MD
Jonas T. Johnson, MD

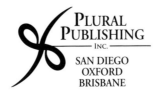

PLURAL
PUBLISHING
INC.
SAN DIEGO
OXFORD
BRISBANE

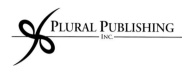

5521 Ruffin Road
San Diego, CA 92123

e-mail: info@pluralpublishing.com
Web site: http://www.pluralpublishing.com

49 Bath Street
Abingdon, Oxfordshire OX14 1EA
United Kingdom

Library of Congress Cataloging-in-Publication Data:

Tracheotomy : airway management, communication, and swallowing / [edited by]
Eugene N. Myers and Jonas T. Johnson. — 2nd ed.
     p. ; cm.
  Includes bibliographical references and index.
  ISBN-13: 978-1-59756-101-3 (pbk.)
  ISBN-10: 1-59756-101-0 (pbk.)
  1. Tracheotomy. 2. Trachea—Surgery. I. Myers, Eugene N., 1933- II.
Johnson, Jonas T.
  [DNLM: 1. Tracheotomy. 2. Tracheostomy. WF 490 T7591 2007]
  RF516.T74 2007
  617.5'33—dc22

                                            2007005292

CONTENTS

SECTION III. REHABILITATION

PREFACE
to the First Edition

Tracheotomy: Airway Management, Communication, and Swallowing is prepared by a multidisciplinary team of health care professionals emphasizing the important issues critical to management of this seemingly simple procedure. Tracheotomy does, in fact, have the potential to be a lifesaving intervention, but it also has profound effects on speech, swallowing, and pulmonary function.

This text has been prepared to reflect the complex physiologic functions affected by tracheotomy. We emphasize the contributions of a variety of health care professionals. It is essential that health care providers caring for tracheotomy patients be expert in these issues.

This era of health care reform has placed great emphasis upon early discharge from hospital and provision of outpatient care to a wide variety of patients. This includes those with tracheotomy. Health care providers must be aware of the impact of tracheotomy upon communication and deglutition. A variety of strategies are available to maximize functional performance under these circumstances. The health care team must also be cognizant of the potential for complications, and strategies for the prevention of these complications; they must be prepared to recognize and treat them.

This text is designed to provide the material necessary to support safe, effective intervention in a variety of both inpatient and outpatient settings, with the hope that it will result in improved care of patients with tracheotomy.

PREFACE
to the Second Edition

Tracheostomy can be the simplest or the most difficult operation that the surgeon is confronted with. This book deals with this operation, and the broader topic of management of the airway, a problem that confronts many different specialties. Tracheostomy played a major role in the management of acute inflammatory disease of the upper airway in the days when diphtheria and H.influenza epiglottitis produced airway obstruction. As these diseases were brought under control by vaccination and antibiotics, the need for tracheostomy for acute airway distress has decreased.

In recent years, there has been a great increase in the use of tracheostomy in patients with more chronic conditions. This includes patients who require ventilatory assistance in order to provide access to the tracheobronchial tree for deep suctioning. The use of long-term tracheostomy has raised many issues having to do with the patient's ability to swallow and to communicate. Accordingly, in the second edition, we have added chapters on communication options and management of swallowing problems.

We are indebted to our excellent group of contributing authors. We believe this second edition fills an important need that is not addressed in a comprehensive manner elsewhere.

We acknowledge the important and cheerful help of Jackie Lynch, our Editorial Coordinator. We also appreciate the support of Dr. Sadanand Singh, the President of Plural Publishing, for his unwavering support over the two editions of this book.

ABOUT THE EDITORS

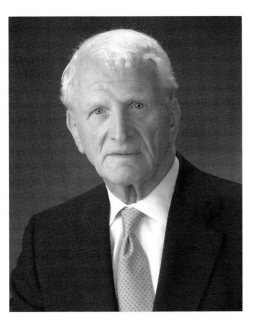

Eugene N. Myers, MD, FACS, FRCS, Edin. (Hon)

Dr. Myers is Distinguished Professor and Emeritus Chair of the Department of Otolaryngology at the University of Pittsburgh School of Medicine. He is internationally recognized as a leader in the field of head and neck surgery. He was Principal Investigator of the Oral Cavity Cancer Center of Discovery sponsored by the National Institute of Dental and Craniofacial Research (NIH). This was funded for $11,000,000 over a 5-year period.

Dr. Myers served as President of the American Board of Otolaryngology, the American Academy of Otolaryngology-Head and Neck Surgery, the American Society of Head and Neck Surgery, the American Laryngological Association and the Pan American Association of Otolaryngology-Head and Neck Surgery. He is an Honorary Fellow of the Royal College of Surgeons of Edinborough and the National Societies of 20 countries.

Dr. Myers served as Coordinator for International Affairs of the American Academy of Otolaryngology-Head and Neck Surgery and was International Editor of Otolaryngology-Head and Neck Surgery. He is a member of the Editorial Board of the *AMA Archives of Otolaryngology-Head and Neck Surgery*, *Head and Neck*, and 13 international journals. *Cancer of the Head and Neck* (4th ed, Elsevier) coauthored with James Y. Suen, MD is considered a classic in the field. He is co-editor of the book *Salivary Gland Disorders* (Springer) with Robert L. Ferris, MD, PhD. He is also Editor of *Otolaryngology-Head and Neck Surgery* (2nd ed, Elsevier).

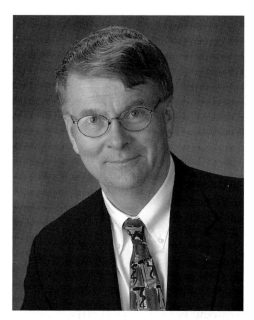

Jonas T. Johnson, MD

Jonas T. Johnson is professor of otolaryngology at the University of Pittsburgh School of Medicine where he holds a joint appointment as professor of Radiation Oncology. He is also professor of oral maxillofacial surgery in the School of Dental Medicine. Dr. Johnson limits his clinical practice to the treatment of patients with tumors of the head and neck as well as the diagnosis and therapy of snoring and obstructive sleep apnea.

Dr. Johnson serves as chairman of the Department of Otolaryngology where he is also the Residency Program Director.

He is presently the Eugene N. Myers, M.D., Chair in Otolaryngology.

Dr. Johnson was an undergraduate at Dartmouth College. He earned his medical degree at SUNY Upstate Medical Center. He later completed his residency at the same institution.

Dr. Johnson has developed his research around the care of patients with cancer of the head and neck. He has special interest and expertise in the management of patients with carcinoma of the upper aerodigestive tract as well as neoplasia of the salivary apparatus and thyroid surgery. He has a major interest in the management of cervical metastasis, surgical therapy for early laryngeal cancer, and adjuvant therapy for advanced head and neck cancer. In 1980, a prospective database of all patients treated for head and neck cancer was established at the University of Pittsburgh. This allowed for an extended period of practice-based learning, which resulted in the publications of over 340 manuscripts in the peer-reviewed literature. Additionally, Dr. Johnson has contributed 144 chapters to textbooks and edited or co-edited 17 texts.

Dr. Johnson is a past president of the American Academy of Otolaryngology–Head and Neck Surgery (2003) and the American Head and Neck Society (2004). He currently serves as editor of the *Laryngoscope*.

CONTRIBUTORS

Lee M. Akst, MD
Assistant Professor
Director, Section of Laryngology
Loyola University Stitch, School of
    Medicine
Maywood, Illinois
Chapter 1

Matthew S. Broadhurst, MD, FRACS
Department of Surgery
Harvard Medical School
Center for Laryngeal Surgery and Voice
    Rehabilitation
Massachusetts General Hospital
Boston, Massachusetts
Chapter 1

Ricardo L. Carrau, MD, FACS
Professor
Medical Director of UPMC Swallowing
    Disorders Center
Department of Otolaryngology
Department of Neurological Surgery
University of Pittsburgh, School of
    Medicine
Pittsburgh, Pennsylvania
Chapter 12

**Karen J. Dikeman MA, CCC-SLP,
BRS-S**
Assistant Vice President
Rehabilitation Services
The Silvercrest Center for Nursing and
    Rehabilitation
Briarwood, New York
Chapter 11

Andrea R. Fox, MD, MPH
Medical Director, Squirrel Hill Health
    Center
Associate Professor of Medicine
University of Pittsburgh, School of
    Medicine
Pittsburgh, Pennsylvania
Chapter 10

Andrew Herlich, DMD, MD, FAAP
Chairman
Department of Anesthesiology
Mercy Hospital of Pittsburgh
Pittsburgh, Pennsylvania
Chapter 2

**Margaret M. Hickey, RN, MSN, MS,
OCN, CORLN**
Associate Director
Clinical Affairs-Oncology
Ortho Biotech Products, L.P.
LaPlace, Louisiana
Chapter 9

**Marilyn Hudak, RN, BSN, MS,
CORLN**
Director, Head and Neck Surgical
    Oncology
Department of Nursing
University of Pittsburgh, Medical Center
Pittsburgh, Pennsylvania
Chapter 9

Jonas T. Johnson, MD
Professor and Chairman
Deptartment of Otolaryngology

Eye and Ear Institute
University of Pittsburgh School of
  Medicine
Pittsburgh, Pennsylvania
Chapter 8

**Marta S. Kazandjian, MA, CCC-SLP,
BRS-S**
Director
Speech Pathology and Swallowing
  Center
New York Hospital Queens
Silvercrest Center for Nursing and
  Rehabilitation
New York, New York
Chapter 11

Karen M. Kost, MD, FRCS(C)
Assistant Professor of Otolaryngology
Director, Voice Laboratory
McGill University
Director of Otolaryngology
Montreal General Hospital
Montreal, Canada
Chapter 5

Carl-Eric Lindholm, MD, PhD
Professor Emeritus of Laryngology and
  Bronchology
Deptartment of Otolaryngology
Uppsala University, School of Medicine
Uppsala, Sweden
Chapter 6

Gerardo Lopez-Guerra, MD
Department of Surgery
Harvard Medical School
Center for Laryngeal Surgery and Voice
  Rehabilitation
Massachusetts General Hospital
Boston, Massachusetts
Chapter 1

Eugene N. Myers, MD
Distinguished Professor and Emeritus
  Chair

Department of Otolaryngology
University of Pittsburgh, School of
  Medicine
Pittsburgh, Pennsylvania
Chapter 3

David A. Nace, MD, MPH
Assistant Professor of Medicine
Director of Long Term Care and Flu
  Programs
University of Pittsburgh Institute on
  Aging
Chief of Medical Affairs
UPMC Senior Living
Pittsburgh, Pennsylvania
Chapter 10

Harvey Slater, MD, FACS
Clinical Professor of Surgery
University of Pittsburgh, School of
  Medicine
Director
Western Pennsylvania Hospital Burn
  Center
Chapter 7

Rohan R. Walvekar, MD
Clinical Assistant Professor
Eye and Ear Institute
Departtment of Otolaryngology-Head
  Neck Surgery
University of Pittsburgh, School of
  Medicine
Pittsburgh, Pennsylvania
Chapter 3

**Tamara Wasserman-Wincko, MS,
CCC-SLP**
Clinical Practice Manager of Speech
  Pathology
Clinical Coordinator of the UPMC
  Swallowing Disorder Center
Clinical Instructor of Otolaryngology
University of Pittsburgh, Medical Center
Pittsburgh, Pennsylvania
Chapter 12

Robert F. Yellon, MD
Associate Professor
Department of Otolaryngology
University of Pittsburgh, School of
  Medicine
Co-Director
Department of Pediatric Otolarynology
Children's Hospital of Pittsburgh
Pittsburgh, Pennsylvania
Chapter 4

Steven M. Zeitels, MD, FACS
Eugene B. Casey Chair of Laryngeal
  Surgery
Department of Surgery, Harvard
  Medical School
Director
Center for Laryngeal Surgery and Voice
  Rehabilitation
Massachusetts General Hospital
Boston, Massachusetts
Chapter 1

To my wife, Barbara, whose patience allowed me to take on the challenge of organizing the second edition of Tracheotomy.

ENM

To the patients who have taught me so much.

JTJ

CHAPTER 1

The History of Tracheotomy and Intubation

STEVEN M. ZEITELS
MATTHEW S. BROADHURST
LEE M. AKST
GERARDO LOPEZ-GUERRA

"Amongst all the operations practiced on man for his relief, I have always thought that 'tracheotomy' should be placed in the first rank which speedily restores to health those who were at the point of death, and thus assimilates the surgeon to the god Esculapius."

Fabricius, 16th century[1]

INTRODUCTION

The tracheotomy procedure was born from the need and desire of physicians to manage and treat ailments and maladies of the respiratory system. This imperative also catalyzed the development of transoral and transnasal intubation. Consequently, there is an inextricable linkage between tracheotomy and endoscopy in the development of these airway procedures, which is especially noteworthy over the past 150 years. Understandably, the evolution of airway management has been influenced by a

This work was supported in part by the Eugene B. Casey Foundation and the Institute of Laryngology and Voice Restoration.

1

number of factors, including (1) understanding of anatomy and physiology, (2) changing disease demographics (ie, infection vs cancer), (3) pharmacology, (4) development of indirect, direct, and flexible laryngoscopy, (5) electricity and illumination, (6) development of organic chemistry to produce better artificial tubes, and (7) instrument and tool-making.

There have been detailed and scholarly explications delineating the development of the tracheotomy procedure from ancient civilizations through the 19th century[1-3] that have been recounted by many subsequent authors in journals and texts. If this subject matter is of keen interest, the reader is encouraged to study these erudite historical investigations and especially that of Antoine Louis (1723–1792).[1] In the present discussion, selected key concepts will be excerpted; however, the emphasis will be on integrating the evolution of transcervical tracheotomy and endoscopic intubation. This latter topic is seldom discussed in detail and has direct applications for the present, providing practical value.

TERMINOLOGY

Transcervical operations to ameliorate airway difficulties have undergone a metamorphosis of vocabulary, which can potentially create confusion. In the 19th century Ryland (1806–1857)[4] and Mackenzie (1837–1892)[5] explained that bronchotomy (seldom used today) is a general term for the various operations by which the air passages are laid open. This includes laryngotomy by means of thyrotomy (separating the thyroid alae),

cricothyroidotomy (opening the cricothyroid membrane), tracheotomy, and tracheostomy. Tracheostomy, as it is frequently used today, is, in fact, inappropriate terminology for the procedure that is typically done. It originally referred to sewing the trachea to the skin, a key advancement in the perfection of total laryngectomy described by Solis-Cohen (1838–1927).[6] Even pharyngotomy has inaccurately been used to describe entering the laryngotracheal airway.

Adding to this confusion is the fact that ancient records of tracheotomy are sometimes vague and do not report enough anatomic detail to retrospectively categorize them easily into our current classification schema. Despite the changing terminology used throughout the text, it is clear that the surgeons in each time period who helped to advance acceptance of tracheotomy had an excellent understanding of the work that had been done many years (or even centuries) before.

ANCIENT CIVILIZATION THROUGH THE MIDDLE AGES AND BEYOND

Tracheotomy has been the sole form of mechanical airway restoration during most of human history. The concept of transoral/transnasal intubation would occur during the past two centuries. The story of tracheotomy is one of changing attitudes toward the procedure and changing indications. From the early history of tracheotomy down through modern times there has been a slowly increasing acceptance of the procedure. Tracheotomy was very rarely performed in ancient times; however, in the last few centuries the reluctance of the medical community to perform tracheotomy gradually gave way to acceptance. Eventually strong support for the procedure developed as surgeons realized the benefits that tracheotomy could provide.

There are predynastic Egyptian tablets that many interpret as the earliest images of tracheotomy which date from about 3600 BC.[7] The *Rig Veda*, a Hindu text, gives a clear description of entering the anterior neck and trachea.[8] The Greek author Homer (~850 BC) makes a reference to tracheotomy in a poem where there is a description of incising the trachea to save a person who was choking.

In the 4th century BC, Alexander the Great (356-323 BC) is said to have performed a tracheotomy with the tip of his sword on a soldier who was choking.[9] Hippocrates (460-375 BC) recognized the need for acute intervention when encountering upper airway obstruction.

> . . . when the eyes are affected and prominent, as in those who are strangled; the face, the gullet, and the neck are on fire though nothing can be seen on inspection. . . . In this case a pipe should be introduced into the throat to admit air into the lungs (Hippocrates).[1]

The first actual named surgeon to perform an elective, nonemergency tracheotomy was Asclepaides (124-56 BC). This description was recorded by Galen (130-200 AD). However, tracheotomy was condemned by most at the time because it was believed that incisions into tracheal cartilage could not heal, thereby negating any benefit to the patient.[1] The Greek surgeon, Antyllus (~250 AD) also was an early advocate of tracheotomy to relieve obstruction from enlarged adenoids and tonsillar as well as certain oral diseases. Centuries later, Paul of Aegina (625-690) acknowledged Antyllus' contribution and provided clear descriptions of the procedure and became one of the early supporters of the operation.[1]

The first documented case of tracheotomy clearly described as "successful" was performed by an Italian physician, Antonio Musa Brasavola (1490-1554).[7] Although he may not have physically performed a tracheotomy, Fabricius (1537-1619) advocated for bronchotomy and the use of a vertical incision to retract the anatomic structures (ie, anterior jugular veins) to expose the airway. He also described placing a cannula-tube to prevent aspiration of the cannula during deep inspiration.[1] The tube was to have (phalanges) wings between the cartilage rings.

His pupil and successor Julius Casserius (1545-1605) did perform tracheotomies and was also active in writing on the subject. His published sketch of the procedure is one of the most famous in head and neck surgery (Fig 1-1). These physicians, and most of those who followed over the next ~300 years, performed what our current conception is of a tracheotomy; however, the terminology that was used was bronchotomy or laryngotomy. During the time of Casserius, more physicians actually performed the procedure than in earlier eras, but many continued to write on the subject without physically performing the procedure.

Nicolas Habicot (1550-1624) made substantial contributions to the use of transcervical airway intervention with multiple cases reported in 1620. He provided the first detailed accounts of suc-

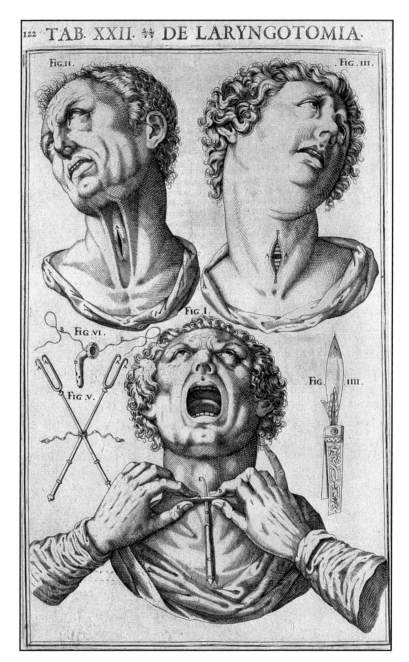

Fig 1–1. Demonstration of a tracheotomy by Julius Casserius from the 16th century.

cessful relief of airway obstruction caused by penetrating neck trauma and a foreign body.[1] In 1694, Dekkers (1648-1720) introduced the concept of percutaneous tracheotomy with a trocar.[1,2] This innovation was noted by other surgeons of the day, causing much debate between people such as Louis,[1] who embraced the use of a trocar and said that the "*operation is greatly simplified by it.*" This 18th century discussion is reminiscent of the academic debate today about percutaneous tracheotomy.[10,11]

It was in this slowly building atmosphere of acceptance that Heister (1683-1758) introduced the term "*tracheotomy*" in 1739 and boldly suggested that his contemporaries should be more aggressive in their use of the procedure.[3] Following his arguments for the more liberal use of tracheotomy, Heister described his own case of tracheotomy in which he extracted an aspirated mushroom from a patient who was at "*danger of suffocation.*" In 1765, Home (1719-1813)[12] described an upper airway inflammation that he called croup, which was an old Scottish word for a sore throat associated with harsh breathing. This term was not widely adopted until well into the 19th century, but remains as a standard term in our vocabulary today.

In his *Memoir on Bronchotomy* in the late 18th century, Louis[1] argues very strongly in favor of tracheotomy: "*No relief can be more prompt than bronchotomy, in a case that requires it.*" He states that the procedure should be performed early in cases of impending airway obstruction rather than done as a last resort. Beyond his own arguments, which also debate the use of tracheotomy in drowning and the use of a trocar, Louis offers an exhaustive account of the history of tracheotomy from Asclepiades through the 1700s. Louis views the evolving acceptance of tracheotomy as a progression from one generation to the next. He indicates his own role in this progression in very straightforward terms, remarking that

"*the fruit of our inquiries will be perhaps for the future to inspire as much confidence [in tracheotomy] as there has been fear hitherto.*"[1]

The story of the death of George Washington (1732-1799) as related by Green[13] and Frost,[8] reveals the atmosphere of trepidation which surrounded tracheotomy in that era. On December 10, 1799, after having been exposed to rain and cold, Washington awoke in his Mount Vernon home with a severe sore throat, hoarseness, odynophagia, and fever. This soon progressed to a feeling of tightness in his throat with labored breathing and stridor. Against his family's urging, Washington initially refused to send for his physician and instead he "*procured a bleeder in the neighborhood.*"[13] On the following day, his physicians, Drs. James Craik and Gustavus Brown, were summoned and he was diagnosed first with quinsy and then with "cynanche trachealis" (croup); recent historians suggest that he was suffering from epiglottitis.[14] They recommended further bleeding, administration of two moderate doses of calomel as a purgative and inhalation of vapours of vinegar and water. These interventions had no effect and his symptoms quickly progressed. As Washington's breathing deteriorated, another physician, Dr. Elisha Dick was summoned. Although Dick recommended tracheotomy, the senior physicians refused and instead continued to bleed President Washington. They removed a total of almost 2.5 L of blood[15] and Washington soon succumbed. Although it unfortunately was of no use for Washington, soon thereafter in the early 19th century, there was increased acceptance and support for tracheotomy as a lifesaving intervention for infectious diseases of the larynx and trachea.

THE PAST 200 YEARS

During the last 2 centuries, the use of tracheotomy increased and the indications broadened corresponding to a number of advances in medicine, surgery, and anesthesia. However, these developments cannot be properly considered without considering the commensurate increase in the use of transoral/transnasal endotracheal intubation. This choice of airway access became especially pertinent as the field of Laryngology was instituted (~1857) with the associated advancing techniques of minimally invasive airway surgery and instrumentation. There is value in tracing the omnipresent clinical decision-making in accessing the laryngotracheal airway endoscopically or transcervically as it provides perspective to current surgeons' decision-making.

It is remarkable that, regardless of the access route to the trachea, the general indications for the procedure have remained relatively unchanged in the past 2 centuries. The most common indications for urgent airway intervention are obstruction from inflammation and/or infection, foreign body, and neoplasm. However, trauma to the neck,[4,16-21] caustic mucosal exposures,[22-24] stenosis.[18,20,25] and vocal-fold paralysis[18,20,26,27] were not uncommon. Advancements in resection techniques for tumors of the head and neck also forced surgeons to control the laryngotracheal airway. As to be expected, access to the trachea allowed for removal of mucopurulent secretions and delivery of pharmacologic agents including anesthesia. Over time, access to the airway allowed progression from brief human-to-human artificial respiration to mechanical ventilation for anesthesia and critical care

management. These thematic indications for accessing the trachea allow for the optimal review of this complex historical development and the interdependence of the advancements.

Airway Obstruction

As described earlier, the origin and primary indication for tracheotomy has always been infectious diseases of the airway, which dates back thousands of years. These diseases have had a wide variety of names including phthisis, cynanche laryngeal, quinsy, laryngeal and pharyngeal angina, diphtheria, consumption, and croup. From ancient civilizations through the 19th century, the procedure was seldom done due to skepticism and limited understanding of human physiology and the biology of these diseases. However, in the earlier 1800s, there was a substantial expansion of investigations and reporting on these diseases. Bretonneau[28,29] (1778–1862), Ryland (1806–1857),[30] Trousseau (1801–1867),[31-33] and Green (1802–1866)[34-39] championed this effort. All were focused on surgical intervention of the larynx and trachea to avert the morbid and frequently fatal complications of these diseases; however, Green was substantially more focused on transoral instrumentation with topical administration of caustics to the diseased laryngotracheal mucous membranes (Fig 1–2).

Despite the expanding acceptance and performance of tracheotomy in the 19th century, it continued to be appropriately perceived by most clinicians as a heroic procedure to be done in dire circumstances, often when the patient was already in extremis. This was especially

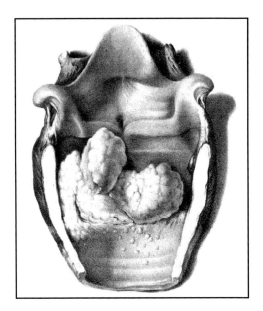

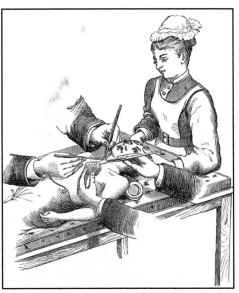

Fig 1–2. Ehrman's depiction of a post-mortem larynx in a patient who died from an exophytic infectious lesion of the laryngeal introitus. It was most likely untreated papillomatosis.[84]

Fig 1–3. Pediatric tracheotomy being performed.

so for those attempting tracheotomy in children. Having successfully performed the first total laryngectomy for cancer,[40] Billroth (1829–1894) provides a compelling description of a 6-year-old child, one of 12. laryngotomy/tracheotomy procedures (Fig 1-3) he reported for treating croup in children.[41]

> This is the only case in which a patient has ever died immediately under the knife at my hands. It made a great and permanent impression on my mind, and has been to me a most decided warning against ever attempting tracheotomy again when single-handed.

Intraprocedural bleeding was commonplace during tracheotomy due to the thyroid gland and anterior jugular veins. If excessive blood was aspirated into the trachea and/or the patient was

exhausted and unable to expectorate ominous circumstances ensued. The surgeon would frequently be required to place a catheter into the airway and clear the trachea by personally suctioning the blood and purulence with his own mouth.[33,41-43] Even today, thoracic surgeons will similarly pass a flexible bronchoscope to aspirate blood and debris on surgical patients.

The majority of patients died despite the airway procedure because the underlying systemic disease process had not been reversed.[29,30,33] Furthermore, the postsurgical management was often as problematic as the procedure itself. Surgeons worked diligently to assist the patients who survived and required a tracheotomy tube long term,. Their creativity is illustrated by the ingenious valves for tracheotomy tubes (Fig 1-4), which were designed to facilitate speech. It is clear that today's plastic appliances simply copied these earlier devices.

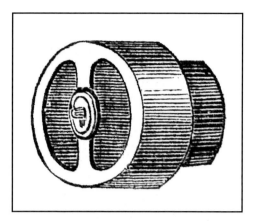 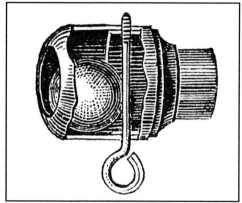

Fig 1–4. Two devices to serve as external appliances for a tracheotomy tube to allow for phonatory function. Notice that the first figure closely resembles a Passy-Muir valve.[68]

As to be expected, most aspects of this management were considerably more problematic in children. Indwelling tubes were not yet perfected and often became occluded and/or dislodged. Adequate lighting was frequently lacking and suction was not yet unavailable. In fact, casts of blood and mucopurulent sloughing membrane had to be removed manually from the trachea by removing the tube. Preoperative and postoperative management could be assisted by a croup tent (Fig 1-5). Ryland,[30] Bretonneau,[29] and Trousseau[33] discussed these issues extensively in their writings. Ryland stated:

> The cannula . . . must be frequently removed and cleansed . . . the medical attendant must be directed to the removal of every obstructing matter the moment that it presents itself. . . . The patient has not the strength enough to project it far, and, consequently, at every inspiration it is sucked again into the trachea, producing in time all the symptoms of impeded respiration, and causing the patient

to sink into an alarming state of disability."[30]

Other sources of upper airway obstruction were various foreign bodies, penetrating and blunt trauma, and caustic exposure. It was routine for surgeons to perform a laryngotomy or tracheotomy to dislodge and/or retrieve obstructing foreign bodies. In 1620, Habicot[3] reported the first tracheotomy used to treat a foreign body. To avoid being robbed, a boy had swallowed his coins, which were wrapped in a cloth and became lodged in his airway. Tracheotmy was discussed extensively over the ensuing centuries by a substantial number of authors including Louis,[1] Ryland,[30] Malgaigne (1806–1865),[43] Gross (1805–1884),[44] Solis Cohen,[45] Mackenzie,[46] and Poulct.[47] A variety of clever instruments[44] were designed to assist with these procedures. In the 20th century, Jackson (1865–1958)[48-50] perfected direct endoscopy of the upper aerodigestive tract which eliminated the need for a tracheotomy in most circumstances.

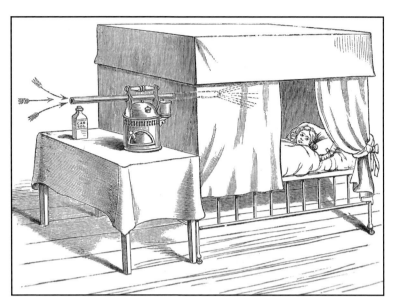

Fig 1–5. Nineteenth century croup tent for child with membranous airway obstruction.

EVOLUTION OF ENDOLARYNGEAL INTUBATION

Endolaryngeal intubation is a relatively recent concept as compared with tracheotomy; however, the indications for both procedures are and have been similar. Both tracheotomy and intubation were conceived to treat and bypass laryngeal and/or pharyngeal airway obstruction. The initial age of development of intubation took place in the 19th century. Instrumenting the endolarynx by way of the natural passages was composed of probangs with distal sponges as well as intubation with catheters to administer pharmacologic agents to diseased aerodigestive tract membranes. Later, tubes were used to protect the airway during resections of tumors of the head and neck. Over time, endolaryngeal intubation was used to enhance access to the tracheobronchial tree for pulmonary toilet as well as to facilitate artificial ventilation during cardiopulmonary resuscitation, normal general endotracheal anesthesia, and critical-care pulmonary management.

Possibly the earliest description of endolaryngeal intubation was by Avicenna (980–1037), who bent tubes of gold and silver to cannulate the larynx and trachea for patients with airway distress. In the late 18th century, Desault (1744–1795),[8,51,52] who was the Surgeon in Chief of the Great Hospital of the Humanity in Paris, revived intubation and described passing a nasotracheal tube to secure the airway. He also was skilled in open transcervical operative techniques and is probably the first surgeon to stress the importance of surgeons retaining skill-sets in transoral and open surgical methods. Desault's technique was well known at the time and described in the famous surgical text by Malgaigne.[52] A century later, this philosophy was more firmly established by Solis-Cohen who was probably the first surgeon to specialize as a Laryngologist.[53]

Green,[34,35,37,39,54] who was the first specialized airway surgeon in the United States, championed the transoral endolaryngeal administration of topical treatment of infectious membranous airway diseases (Fig 1–6). He used a whalebone probang with a distal sponge (Fig 1–7) as well as catheters for this purpose. He also performed the first direct laryngoscopy and visually controlled endoscopic excision of a laryngeal neoplasm, which was done in a young girl, who had airway obstruction from a ball-valving polyp.[36] Bouchut (1818–1891)[55,56] also

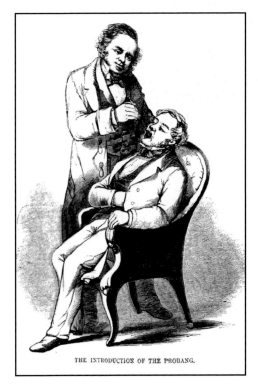

THE INTRODUCTION OF THE PROBANG.

Fig 1–6. Horace Green performing blind orotracheal cannulation of the larynx and trachea with a whalebone probang to administer topical silver nitrate to the diseased membranes of the airway.[94]

was adept at treating croup transorally. After the technique of mirror laryngoscopy[57-59] was formally adopted, nasotracheal and orotracheal catheterization for laryngeal airway obstruction was facilitated by visual guidance.[60]

Regardless of whether surgeons adopted a transoral/transnasal approach (ie, Green) or tracheotomy (ie, Ryland, Trousseau) to remedy airway obstruction, infectious membranous airway maladies created a medical and surgical imperative to access and treat the diseased mucosa. Topical pharmacologic agents such as silver nitrate or mercurial compounds were mainstays of treatment in the 19th century and the aforementioned airway interventions also provided a route of administration for delivering these agents. However, these topical agents did not treat the underlying disorder, which is why mortality rates remained high despite successful airway palliation.

Despite a range of systemic pharmacologic treatment strategies leading to successful management of most infectious airway ailments in the 20th century, aggressive recurrent respiratory papillomatosis remains as the 21st-century vestige of this era as systemic control remains disappointing. To combat this potentially obstructing mucosal disease (see Fig 1–2), fiber-based laser technologies[61,62] are used currently instead of topical pharmacologic agents and advancements in distal-chip flexible endoscope technology have enhanced identification and delivery of the laser to the target tissue.

O'Dwyer (1841–1898)[63-65] was not the first to intubate the larynx for obstruction and infectious disease but he is certainly the individual most responsible for establishing a reliable approach, designing novel instrumentation (Fig 1–8), standardizing the tech-

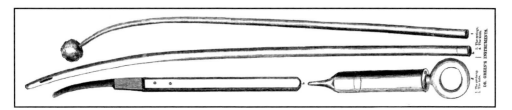

Fig 1–7. Green's instruments for laryngotracheal topical treatment; a whalebone probang with a distal sponge and a syringe-cannula for administration of topical fluid caustics to treat the diseased tracheobronchial membranes.[94]

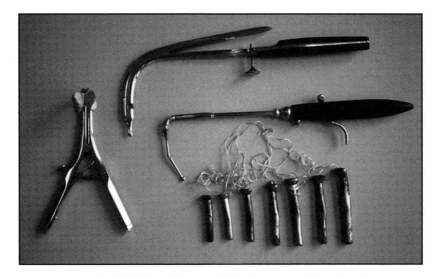

Fig 1–8. An O'Dwyer intubating cannula set.

nique, and establishing its validity. Remarkably, this was a tactile blind approach in children (Fig 1-9) who would not cooperate with mirror laryngoscopy. Similar to Green's experience, the procedure was feasible due to the favorable cephalad position of the larynx in the pediatric population.

O'Dwyer's work was extensive and represented a major paradigm shift as tracheotomy was a well-established standard of care by the late 19th century. However, the opportunity for this advancement was ever present due to the overall mortality of these diseases despite successful airway intervention and because tracheotomy in the pediatric population was perceived as a morbid and dangerous procedure. The subsequent literature was replete with discussions comparing the advantages and disadvantages of intubation and tracheotomy. Over time, diphtheria antitoxin, direct laryngoscopic intubation, and mechanical ventilation diminished the controversy. However, patients who are expected to have long-term mechanical ventilation still require a decision as to when a tracheotomy should be performed to diminish the trauma to the larynx associated with oral-nasal endotracheal intubation.

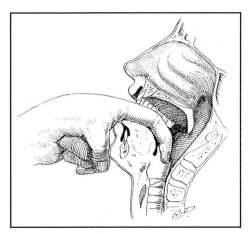
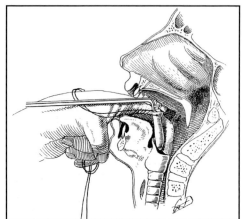
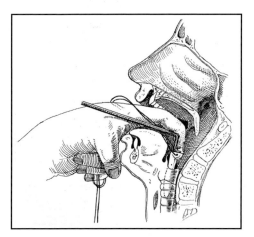
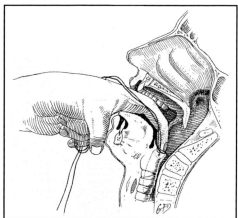

Fig 1–9. Detailed illustration of the O'Dwyer technique for blind and manual placement of a cannula in a pediatric patient suffering from airway obstruction.

Intratracheal Anesthesia

Intratracheal anesthesia has undergone a metamorphosis in the past 200 years. Bigelow (1818–1890)[66] reported on Morton's (1819–1868) administration of ether anesthesia for Warren's (1778–1856) resection of a benign neck mass at the Massachusetts General Hospital in 1846. Soon thereafter, the tracheotomy cannula was used as a direct portal for intratracheal anesthesia.

Trendelenburg (1844–1924)[67-69] devised a tracheotomy tube with a cuff (Fig 1–10) to prevent blood from entering the trachea, which was the precursor of modern closed-system endotracheal anesthesia.

It is likely that Macewen (1848–1924)[70] was the first to intubate the patient transorally for anesthetic purposes, which was done for an extensive resection of the oral cavity/oropharynx. Chloroform was administered and the lower pharynx

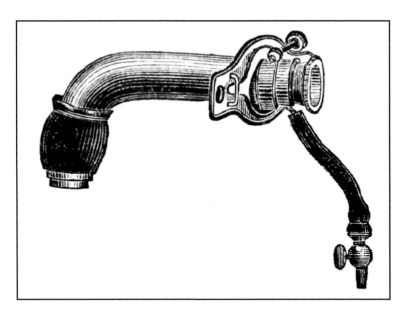

Fig 1–10. Semon's modification of Trendelenburg's tracheotomy tube which was fitted with a distal cuff to preclude blood from being aspirated into the distal tracheobronchial tree during neoplasm resections of the oral cavity and pharynx.[68]

was packed to seal the airway and to inhibit blood from the resection being aspirated. This patient underwent a mandibulotomy for access to the neoplasm with subsequent wiring of the mandibular segments and extubation. In 1889, Annandale (1839-1908)[24] introduced a new orotracheal tube and reported that he intubated several patients transorally to treat a variety of problems to control the airway and to administer anesthesia. This included a large thyroid cancer, a deep-neck-space infection, and a caustic mucosal burn in a child.

Shortly after its discovery,[71] Kirstein (1863-1922)[72,73] used topical cocaine anesthesia to facilitate direct laryngoscopy and tracheoscopy (1895) while formally introducing the technique. It is surprising that this innovation was not rapidly incorporated into general inhalation anesthesia. (Fig 1-11) In fact, Kuhn (1866-1929)[74,75] combined concepts from O'Dwyer's tube and Trendelenburg's cannula into his orotracheal intubation system (Fig 1-12) for anesthesia. He employed a malleable metal tube that would be blindly passed through the glottis and could be fitted with an assortment of balloons that could tamponade the pharynx, laryngeal introitus, or trachea. Remarkably, Kuhn's device is reminiscent of the coiled metal that comprises flexible endoscopes, which were introduced in 1957 by Hirschowitz (1925).[76,77]

Meltzer (1851-1920) and Auer (1875-1948)[78] experimented further with Kuhn' insufflation techniques in an experimental setting. Soon thereafter in 1910, Elsberg (1871-1948), a pioneering neurosurgeon, introduced these methods clinically, which ushered in the

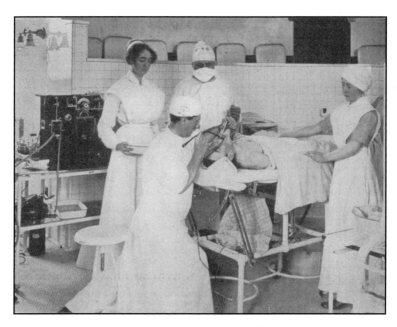

Fig 1–11. An early 20th century photograph of a patient being catheterized for insufflation anesthesia.[95]

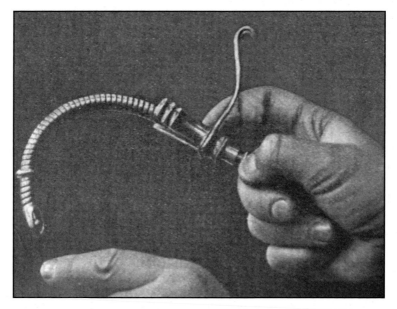

Fig 1–12. The Kuhn articulating malleable intubation tube, which was used without direct visualization.[74]

modern era of direct orotracheal intubation and general endotracheal anesthesia. Elsberg[79,80] was assisted by Yankauer (1872–1932) who had learned direct laryngoscopic techniques from Jackson.[81]

Artificial Respiration

Tracheotomy allowed for control of the airway which led to the concept of mechanical artificial respiration.[4,42] Ryland[4] explained that apart from airway obstruction and removal of a foreign body, a crucial indication for endotracheal catheterization and bronchotomy was to facilitate the performance of artificial respiration in cases of suspended animation. Similar to today, patients could require this intervention for drowning or substance abuse.

> Tracheotomy may also be required during the insensibility produced by taking large quantities of ardent spirits or the narcotic poisons, as opium and prussic acid. In such cases artificial respiration is sometimes rendered necessary by the prostration of the whole muscular energies and consequently of those of the respiratory muscles; and in the absence of a proper tube for introduction into the glottis by way of the nostril, an opening must be made into the larynx or trachea, to allow for the insertion of the pipe of the bellows.[4]

As surgeons acquired a greater experience with tracheotomy in the 1800s, they developed an enhanced comfort level with the procedure and its postoperative management. Given the increasing frequency of tracheotomy, it was not uncommon for some patients to have bleeding into the airway and/or to cease respiration due to the underlying condition that precipitated the need for the airway intervention.[4,41,82] If patients became obtunded from the collection of tracheobronchial fluid the airway lumen was cleared, and the surgeon would then commence artificial respiration by blowing air into the trachea by means of a catheter or tube.

In the 20th century, the concepts for positive-pressure insufflation anesthesia, cardiopulmonary resuscitation, and critical-care mechanical ventilation were fully developed. The efficacy of these techniques was enhanced by widespread adoption of direct-laryngoscopic techniques with improved endotracheal tubes, a range of pharmacologic agents for general anesthesia, the advent of critical-care medicine, and sophisticated understanding of cardiopulmonary physiology.

Intratracheal Intubation for Neoplasms of the Head and Neck

The first publicized procedure using general anesthesia was done for a mass in the neck.[66] By this time, tracheotomy had gained greater acceptance and was becoming commonplace. These advances provided unique and expanding possibilities for resecting neoplasms of the head and neck. The procedures can be stratified into laryngeal resections and pharynx/oral-cavity excisions. After initially failing, Ehrman (1792–1878)[83,84] performed a laryngotomy for cannula placement to treat laryngeal airway obstruction and a secondary staged successful laryngofissure to resect a benign obstructing laryngeal neoplasm (see Fig 1–2). Green[85] credits Ehrman for providing him with the inspiration to attempt direct laryngoscopy.

Tracheotomy became more accepted as a universal therapeutic intervention for upper airway distress in the prelaryngology (before 1857) era prior to widespread adoption of mirror laryngoscopy. Tracheotomy was often used to bypass a variety of obstructing benign and malignant laryngeal and pharyngeal neoplasms. Due to the hazards of extensive upper aerodigestive tract tumor resections, tracheotomy continued as a common palliative therapeutic intervention well into the late 19th century even though clinicians could visualize (mirror laryngoscopy) neoplasms. The most remarkable of these cases was the Crown Prince Frederick (1831–1888) of Germany[86] who developed an obstructing laryngeal cancer and underwent a therapeutic tracheotomy. Despite the delayed diagnosis, which eventually established the cancer, the Prince's surgeon had limited experience with partial or total laryngectomy. Prince Frederick became Emperor for the last 90 days of his life, which was facilitated by the tracheotomy. Had he undergone the cancer resection, he would have likely died in the perioperative period and never assumed the throne.[87]

In 1851, Buck (1807–1887)[88] performed a cricothyroidotomy for airway stabilization and was the first to perform a laryngofissure in the United States. There is conflicting opinion about whether the lesion excised was a cancer, which relates in part to the state-of-the-art of anatomical pathology at the time (Fig 1–13). Unfortunately, the patient died within the year. Sands (1830–1888)[89] performed a similar procedure on a patient who clearly had cancer. Unfortunately, however, his patient met a similar fate. In 1866, Durham (1833–1895)[90] reported two children in whom a tracheotomy was performed with administration of chloroform followed by a laryngofissure and successful resection of benign obstructing laryngeal lesions. In 1869, Solis-Cohen performed a tracheotomy and hemilaryngectomy for cancer achieving a long-term cure. This patient, who was the son of a professor at the University of

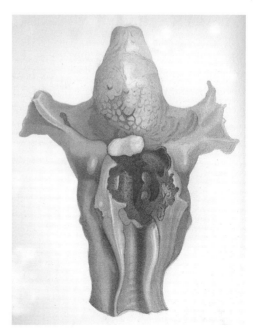

Fig 1–13. The postmortem larynx and trachea of the patient who died after Buck performed the first laryngotomy in America.[88]

Pennsylvania, removed his tracheotomy tube himself after a number of months and survived 20 years. It is likely that this was the first reported cure of a laryngeal cancer.

The use of the tracheotomy made surgery possible by securing the airway to resect neoplasms of the oral cavity and pharynx. An initial tracheotomy allowed for packing the lower pharynx so that blood associated with the excision was not aspirated. Over time, the tracheotomy tube also provided an effective route for administration of inhalation anesthesia. The tracheotomy also protected the upper airway from swelling postoperatively. Taken together, tracheotomy allowed for the safe resection of larger lesions. This approach was espoused by Gross,[91] Sands,[18] and Butlin (1843–1912).[92]

In a seminal article in 1880, Macewen[70] acknowledged tracheotomy as an effective approach to stabilize the airway in upper aerodigestive-tract resections. As an alternative strategy, he boldly intubated transorally a patient who was undergoing a radical resection of a large oropharynx cancer through a mandibulotomy approach. The procedure was quite successful as the hypopharynx packing prevented blood from entering the trachea and chloroform was used successfully as inhalation anesthetic. After successfully using the intubation approach in two more patients for laryngeal edema, a fourth patient died from a chloroform complication during excision of a cancer of the head and neck. It appears that Macewen abandoned the approach after the death of this patient. Kuhn then resurrected the approach with his novel metal transoral tube, which was also used to secure the airway for a resection of cancer of the pharynx and to administer anesthesia.[74] Understandably, tracheotomy remains as a routine component of the resection of a majority of medium to large neoplasms of the oral cavity and pharynx. However, similar to the aforementioned cases, extensive resections in the oropharynx cannot be done without performing a tracheotomy.[93]

SUMMARY

Tracheotomy is one of the oldest surgical procedures recorded in human history. It was born from the omnipresent condition of impending death from airway obstruction. Despite the evolving demographics of diseases and trauma, access to the tracheobronchial lumen will remain an imperative to ensure adequate ventilation. The interdependent development and evolution of transcervical tracheotomy and intubation through the natural passages is a remarkable chronicle of disease, survival, medical and surgical evolution, creative tool-making, and scientific discovery. This narrative parallels and retains essential aspects of the origin and development of minimally invasive surgery as surgeons strive to achieve key therapeutic objectives while diminishing patient morbidity. Tracheal cannulation will always be a crucial element in the management of a wide variety of upper aerodigestive tract maladies. This rich history should provide surgeons with valuable perspectives on their current strategies for airway management.

REFERENCES

1. Louis A. Louis on Bronchotomy. Presentation before the Royal Academy of Surgery of France in 1784. In: *Observations on Surgical diseases of the Head and Neck*. London, UK: New Sydenham Society; 1848:214-278.
2. Wright, J. Tracheotomy. In: *A History of Laryngology and Rhinology*. 2nd ed. Philadelphia Pa: Lea & Febiger; 1914:65, 92, 152-158.
3. Goodall EW. The story of tracheotomy. *Br J Child Dis*. 1934;31:167-176, 253-272.
4. Ryland F. Bronchotomy. In: *Diseases and Injuries of the Larynx and Trachea*. Philadelphia Pa: Carey and Hart; 1841:213-230.
5. Mackenzie M. Bronchotomy, including tracheotomy and (cricothyroid) laryngotomy. In: *Diseases of the Pharynx, Larynx, and Trachea*. New York, NY: William Wood & Co; 1880:396-401.
6. Solis-Cohen J. Two cases of laryngectomy for adeno-carcinoma of the larynx. *Trans Am Laryngo Assoc*. 1892;14:60-67.

7. Sercer A. Tracheotomy through two thousand years of history. *CIBA Symp.* 1962;10:78–86.

8. Frost EA. tracing the tracheotomy. *Ann Otol Rhinol Laryngol.* 1976;85:618–624.

9. Gordon, BL. *The Romance of Medicine.* Philadelphia, Pa: FA Davis; 1947:461.

10. Ciaglia P, Firsching R, Syniec C. Elective percutaneous dilational tracheostomy. A new simple bedside procedure; preliminary report. *Chest.* 1985;87:715–719.

11. Kost KM. Endoscopic percutaneous dilational tracheotomy. A prospective evaluation of 500 consecutive cases. *Chest.* 2005;87:715–719.

12. Home F. *An Enquiry into the Natural Causes and Cure of Croup.* Edinburgh: Kincaid and Bell; 1765.

13. Green H. *A Treatise on Diseases of the Air Passages.* New York, NY: Wiley and Putnam; 1846:32–34.

14. Morens DM. Death of a president. *N Engl J Med.* 1999;341(24):1845–1849.

15. Schmidt PJ., Transfuse George Washington! *Transfusion.* 2002;42(2): 275–277.

16. Adams T. Two remarkable cases in surgery: cut throat injury. *The London Magazine.* 1763, July: 369–370.

17. Gross S. Injuries and diseases of the neck. In: *A System of Surgery.* Philadelphia, Pa: Blanchard & Lea; 1859;382–386.

18. Sands HB. Tracheotomy and laryngotomy. In: *American Clinical Lectures.* 1876:183–222.

19. Solis-Cohen J. Wounds of the larynx and trachea. In: *Diseases of the Throat: A Guide to the Diagnosis and Treatment.* New York, NY: William Wood; 1879:600–607.

20. Mackenzie M. *Diseases of the Pharynx, Larynx, and Trachea.* New York, NY: William Wood & Co; 1880.

21. Billroth T. Laryngotomy and tracheotomy. In: *Clinical Surgery.* London, UK: New Sydenham Society; 1881:141–142.

22. Ryland F. Injuries of the larynx from drinking boiling water and concentrated acids, and from the inhalation of flame, in diseases and injuries of the larynx and

trachea. Philadelphia, Pa: Carey and Hart; 1841:186–196.

23. Gross S. Diseases and injuries of the air-passages: scalds: In: *A System of Surgery.* Philadelphia, Pa: Blanchard & Lea; 1859:356.

24. Annandale T. Intubation of the larynx and air-passages, with a description of a new instrument as an aid to certain operations. *Br Med J.* 1889:463–465.

25. Solis-Cohen J. Chronic laryngitis. In: *Diseases of the Throat: A Guide to the Diagnosis and Treatment.* New York, NY: William Wood; 1872:473–496.

26. Solis-Cohen J. Paralysis of the muscles of the larynx. In: *Diseases of the Throat: A Guide to the Diagnosis and Treatment.* New York, NY: William Wood; 1872: 636–659.

27. Browne L. Neuroses of the larynx. In: *The Throat and Its Diseases.* Philadelphia, Pa: Lea and Febiger; 1878:272–292.

28. Bretonneau P. *Des Inflammations speciales du tissu muqueux et en particulier de la diphtherite, ou inflammation pelliculaire.* Paris, France: Crevot; 1826.

29. Bretonneau P. *Memoirs on Diphtheria from the writings of Breoneau, Guersant, Trousseau, Bouchut, Empis, and Daviot.* London, UK: New Sydenham Society; 1858:1–204.

30. Ryland F. *Diseases and Injuries of the Larynx and Trachea.* Philadelphia, Pa: Carey and Hart; 1841.

31. Trousseau A. Memoire sur un cas de tracheotomie practiquee dansleperiode extreme de croup. *J Connaiss Med Chir.* 1833;1:5, 41.

32. Trousseau A. Belloc H. *Phthisie Laryngie.* Paris, France: Chez and Bailliere; 1837.

33. Trousseau A. Belloc H. *Laryngeal Phthisis, Chronic Laryngitis and Diseases of the Voice.* Philadelphia, Pa: Carey and Hart; 1841.

34. Green H. *A Treatise on Diseases of the Air Passages.* New York, NY: Wiley and Putnam; 1846.

35. Green H. *Observations on the Pathology of Croup*. New York, NY: John Wiley; 1849.

36. Green H. Morbid growths within the larynx, In: *On the Surgical Treatment of Polypi of the Larynx, and Oedema of the Glottis*. New York, NY: GP. Putnam; 1852:46-65.

37. Green H. On the subject of the priority in the medication of the larynx and trachea. *Am Med Monthly*. 1854:241-257.

38. Green H. Remarks on croup and its treatment. *Am Med Monthly*. 1854:401-421.

39. Green H. Report on the use and effect of applications of nitrate silver to the throat, either in local or general disease. *Trans Am Med Assoc*. 1856;9:493-530.

40. Gussenbauer C. Ueber die erste durch Th. Billroth am Menschen, Ausgerfuhrte Kehlkopf Exstirpation und die Anwendungeines kunstlichen Kehlkopfes. *Archiv fur Klinische Chirurgie*. 1874;17:343-356.

41. Billroth T. Thirteen cases of laryngotomy and tracheotomy for laryngeal croup, In: *Clinical Surgery*. London, UK: New Sydenham Society; 1881:139-140.

42. Gross S. Diseases and injuries of the air-passages: bronchotomy. In: *A System of Surgery*. Philadelphia, Pa: Blanchard & Lea; 1859:379-382.

43. Malgaigne JF. Operations on the throat: bronchotomy. In: *Operative Surgery*. Philadelphia, Pa: Blanchard and Lea; 1851:369-372.

44. Gross S. Diseases and injuries of the air-passages: foreign bodies, In: *A System of Surgery*. Philadelphia, Pa: Blanchard & Lea; 1859;362-379.

45. Solis-Cohen J. Foreign bodies in the larynx and trachea, In: *Diseases of the Throat: A Guide to the Diagnosis and Treatment*. New York, NY: William Wood; 1879:614-624.

46. Mackenzie M. Foreign bodies in the trachea, In: *Diseases of the Pharynx, Larynx, and Trachea*. New York, NY: William Wood & Co; 1880:411-417.

47. Poulet A. Expulsion and extraction through artificial channels—tracheotomy and laryngotomy, In: *Treatise on Foreign Bodies in Surgical Practice*. New York, NY: William F Wood; 1880:78-95.

48. Jackson C. *Tracheo-Bronchoscopy, Esophagoscopy and Gastroscopy*. St. Louis, Mo: The Laryngoscope Co; 1907.

49. Jackson C. *Peroral Endoscopy and Laryngeal Surgery*. St. Louis, Mo: The Laryngoscope Co; 1915.

50. Jackson C. Jackson CL. *The Larynx and Its Diseases*. Philadelphia, Pa: WB Saunders; 1937.

51. Bichat X. *The Surgical Works, or State of the Doctrine and Practice of P.J. Desault*. Philadelphia, Pa; Thos Dolson; 1814:229-234.

52. Malgaigne JF. Operations on the throat: catheterism of the air-passages, In: *Operative Surgery*. Philadelphia, Pa: Blanchard and Lea; 1851:368-369.

53. Zeitels SM. Jacob Da Silva Solis-Cohen: America's first head and neck surgeon. *Head Neck*. 1997;19(4):342-346.

54. Green H. *Bronchial Injections: 106 Cases of Pulmonary Diseases*. New York, NY: Edward P. Allen; 1856.

55. Bouchut M. On a new method of treating croup by tubage of the larynx. *Lancet*. 1858:364.

56. Bouchut M. *Memoirs on Diphtheria from the writings of Breoneau, Guersant, Trousseau, Bouchut, Empis, and Daviot*. London, UK: New Sydenham Society; 1859 (translated from original in 1852):271-297.

57. Garcia M. Observations on the human voice. *Proc Roy Soc Lond*. 1855;7:397-410.

58. Czermak JN. Ueber den Kehlkopfspiegel. *Wiener Med Wochenschrift*. 1858;8(13):196-198.

59. Turck L. On the laryngeal mirror and its mode of employment, with engravings on wood. *Zeitschrift der Gesellschaft der Aerzte zu Wien*. 1858:26:401-409.

60. Solis-Cohen J. Catheterization of the larynx and trachea, In: *Diseases of the Throat: A Guide to the Diagnosis and*

Treatment. New York, NY: William Wood; 1879:679-680.

61. Zeitels SM, Franco RA Jr, Dailey SH, et al. Office-based treatment of glottal dysphasia. *Ann Otol Rhinol Laryngol.* 2004;113(4):265-276.

62. Zeitels SM. Office-based 532-nm pulsed KTP laser treatment of glottal papillomatosis and dysplasia. *Ann Otol Rhino Laryngol.* 2006;115:686-689.

63. O'Dwyer J. Intubation of the larynx. *NY Med J.* 1885;42:145-147.

64. O'Dwyer J. Chronic stenosis of the larynx treated by a new method. *NY Med Rec.* 1886;June 5.

65. O'Dwyer J. Fifty cases of croup in private practice treated by intubation of the larynx, with a description of the method and the dangers incident thereto. *Med Rec.* 1887;32:557-561.

66. Bigelow HJ. Insensibility during surgical operations produced by inhalation. *Boston Med Surg J.* 1846:309-317, 379-382.

67. Trendelenburg F. Beitrage zu den Operationen an den Luftwegen. *Arch Klin Chir.* 1871;12:112-133.

68. Mackenzie M. Tracheotomy instruments, In: *Diseases of the Pharynx, Larynx, and Trachea.* New York, NY: William Wood & Co; 1880:373-379.

69. Solis-Cohen J. Morbid growths of the larynx, In: *Diseases of the Throat: A Guide to the Diagnosis and Treatment.* New York, NY: William Wood; 1879:534-576.

70. Macewen W. Introduction to tracheal tubes by the mouth instead of performing tracheotomy or laryngotomy. *Br Med J.* 1880;122-124, 163-165.

71. Jelinek E. Das Cocain als Anastheticum und Analgeticum fur den Pharynx und Larynx. *Wiener Medizinische Wochenschrift.* 1884;34:1334-1337, 1364-1367.

72. Kirstein,A. Autoskopie des Larynx und der Trachea (Laryngoscopia directa, Euthyskopie, Besichtigung ohne Spiegel).

Archiv fur Laryngologie und Rhinologie. 1895;3:156-164.

73. Kirstein A. *Autoscopy of the Larynx and Trachea (Direct Examination Without Mirror).* Philadelphia, Pa: Davis; 1897.

74. Kuhn F. Perorale Tubagen mit und ohne Druck. *Deutsche Zeitschrift fur Chirurgie.* 1905;76:148-207.

75. Kuhn F. Die Perorale Intubation mit ohne Druck. *Deutsche Zeitschrift fur Chirurgie.* 1905;78:477.

76. Hirschowitz BI. Preliminary report on a long fiberscope for examination of the stomach and duodenum. *Univ Michigan Med Bull.* 1957;23:178-180.

77. Hirschowitz BI. A fibre optic flexible oesophagoscope. *Lancet.* 1963:388-398.

78. Meltzer SJ. Auer J. Continuous respiration without respiratory movements. *J Exp Med.* 1909;11:622-625.

79. Elsberg CA. Clinical experiences with intratracheal insufflation [Meltzer], with remarks upon the value of the method for thoracic surgery. *Ann of Surg.* 1910;52:23-29.

80. Elsberg CA. The value of continuous intratracheal insufflation of air [Meltzer] in thoracic surgery. *Med Rec.* 1910:493-495.

81. Jackson C. Direct laryngoscopy, In: *Tracheo-Bronchoscopy, Esophagoscopy and Gastroscopy.* St. Louis, Mo: The Laryngoscope Co; 1907:39-43.

82. Trousseau A. Belloc H. *Laryngeal Phthisis, Chronic Laryngitis and Diseases of the Voice.* Philadelphia, Pa: Carey and Hart; 1841:157.

83. Ehrmann C H. Sur une operation de laryngotomie pratiquee dans un cas de polype du larynx. *C R Acad Sci (Paris).* 1844;18:593, 709.

84. Ehrmann C H. *Histoire des Polyps du Larynx.* Straasbourg; 1854.

85. Green H. *On the Surgical Treatment of Polypi of the Larynx, and Oedema of the Glottis.* New York, NY: G P Putnam; 1852.

86. Mackenzie M. *The Fatal Illness of Frederick the Noble*. London, UK: Sampson, Low, Marston, Searle and Rivington Ltd; 1888.
87. Delavan DB. A consideration of the statistics of the operations for the relief of malignant disease of the larynx. *Trans Am Laryngol Assoc*, 1900;22:66-74.
88. Buck G. On the surgical treatment of morbid growths within the larynx. *Trans Amer Med Assn*. 1853;6:509-535.
89. Sands HB. Case of cancer of the larynx, successfully removed by laryngotomy; with an analysis of 50 cases of tumors of the larynx, treated by operation. *N Y Med J*. 1865:110-126.
90. Durham A E. Operations on the larynx, In: *Guys Hospital Reports*. London, UK; 1866.
91. Gross S. Morbid growths of the pharynx, In: *A System of Surgery*. Philadelphia, Pa; Blanchard & Lea; 1859:249-253.
92. Butlin HT. Excision of the tongue. In: *Diseases of the Tongue*. London: Cassell and Company; 1900.
93. Zeitels SM, Vaughan CW. Ruh S. Suprahyoid pharyngotomy for oropharynx cancer including the tongue base. *Arch Otolaryngol Head Neck Surg*. 1991;117:757-760.
94. Dr. Horace Green and his method. In: *Harper's Weekly*. February 5, 1859: 88-90.
95. Jackson C. Anesthesia for peroral endoscopy. In: *Peroral Endoscopic Laryngeal Surgury*. St. Louis, Mo: The Laryngoscope Co; 1915:54-72.

CHAPTER 2

Alternatives to Tracheostomy

ANDREW HERLICH

Tracheostomy is the surgical alternative when airway compromise cannot be managed by other means. Less invasive means of establishing a patent airway are usually considered prior to performing a tracheostomy. The alternative methods vary from patient to patient, and cannot be universally applied. Practitioners who care for patients requiring airway management and ventilation must be familiar with the varying modalities as well as their indications and contraindications.

NONINVASIVE POSITIVE-PRESSURE VENTILATION

Bag-mask-valve ventilation with facemask and self-inflating resuscitation bag is usually the first choice in patient ventilation. It requires that the mask have an appropriate fit and seal. The practitioner adminis-

tering this type of ventilation must be facile with the technique as it requires constant vigilance. It is not suitable for long periods of time due to practitioner fatigue and the potential risk for aspiration of abdominal contents in the at-risk population. Success of this technique may not be readily achieved in patients with severe facial deformities or injuries. In patients who have a stenotic airway, heliox, a fixed combination of helium and oxygen may improve oxygenation as the gas combination improves laminar flow. Nasopharyngeal and oropharyngeal airways may be important adjuncts in successful bag-mask-valve ventilation especially in the edentulous patient. The very large or morbidly obese patient may require two rescuers for successful ventilation. One rescuer will hold the mask while a second rescuer compresses the resuscitation bag.

Noninvasive positive-pressure ventilation may be successful in certain patients with acute respiratory failure. Except for patients with chronic obstructive pulmonary disease, the suitable candidates must be cooperative and conscious. In the critical care patient population, non-invasive ventilation improves preoxygenation before endotracheal intubation in the hypoxic patient.[1] These patients tend to desaturate more rapidly than patients in the operating room presenting for elective surgery. Unfortunately, the technique is not an appropriate rescue or temporizing modality in patients who have been extubated in the critical care units and require reintubation.[2] Noncandidates include those with facial trauma, recent gastrointestinal surgery, or bleeding in the gastrointestinal tract. Cardiovascular instability is also an important contraindication to the technique.

SUPRAGLOTTIC VENTILATION

The American Society of Anesthesiologists has a suggested algorithm for management of the difficult airway.[3] However, the algorithm also applies to the routine airway. Included in the algorithm is an example of a supraglottic airway, the laryngeal mask airway. Developed by Dr. Archie Brain, it is simple to insert, passed blindly without auxiliary devices, and has a low frequency of complications. A number of manufacturers have developed slightly different versions of this device. In general, the standard laryngeal mask airway does not protect against aspiration of abdominal contents. A version of the laryngeal mask airway, the Proseal™ Laryngeal Mask Airway has a gastric port which permits passage of a stomach tube but does not afford the level of airway protection again aspira-

tion that is associated with an endotracheal tube.

The laryngeal mask airway has been modified in several versions to facilitate intubation of the trachea, tracheal visualization during placement, and a flexible version that facilitates head and neck surgery. The Fastrach™ laryngeal mask (also called an intubating laryngeal mask) airway is fashioned around a hollow tube and has a handle to assist in placement. Once in place, a special endotracheal tube may be blindly passed through its lumen into the trachea. On confirmation of endotracheal tube placement with auscultation and capnography, the Fastrach™ laryngeal mask airway may be removed. The Fastrach™ has been well established as a rescue device in difficult airways.[4] The C-Trach™ is the laryngeal mask airway that is attached to a camera that enables the practitioner to see the glottic opening and pass an endotracheal tube under direct vision in circumstances of difficult intubation. The popularity of this device is limited by the expense associated with all airway devices that have cameras (Fig 2–1).

The Combitube™ and King Laryngeal Tracheal Device are also placed blindly without laryngoscopes or other similar instruments. In a study of their use by Army combat medic students, it was shown that both are relatively easy to place on the first attempt, requiring minimal time, less than 25 seconds and 12 seconds, respectively.[5] The Combitube™ has both an esophageal lumen and tracheal lumen with a pharyngeal cuff and distal cuff to permit tracheal ventilation while minimizing the risk of tracheal aspiration. The King LT™ is a single lumen, dual cuff device that occludes the proximal oropharynx and obturates the distal end of the lumen in an attempt to occlude

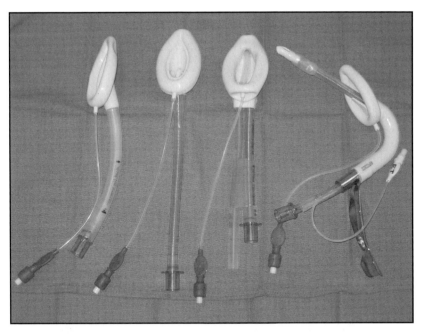

Fig 2–1. Laryngeal mask airways.

the esophagus. Blind intubation of the trachea with the King LT™ is extremely rare. In a recent study of its ease of insertion and function by anesthesiologists, it was found to be fast, simple, and reliable.[6] The Cobra Perilaryngeal Airway (PLA) is another supraglottic airway that is designed to obturate the oropharynx without glottic or tracheal entry. When compared to a laryngeal mask airway for time of insertion, oxygen saturation, and technical difficulty, they were all similar[7] (Figs 2-2 and 2-3).

SUBGLOTTIC INVASIVE VENTILATION

The most frequent form of invasive ventilation is endotracheal intubation. The endotracheal tube may be placed by three routes using numerous techniques. The oral route of tracheal intubation is the most widely used and easiest to perform of the three. It is also the route that has the least adverse outcomes aside from esophageal intubation. Although the oral endotracheal tube may be placed digitally or blindly, use of a rigid or flexible fiberoptic laryngoscope is the most common means of facilitating orotracheal intubation. Depending upon the circumstances, the clinician may chose to use a stylet to maintain rigidity of the tube. On very rare occasions, the orotracheal tube may be placed via a retrograde technique.

Nasotracheal intubation is an alternative but no less important technique that facilitates protection of the airway. Nasotracheal intubation has the advantage of avoiding the oral cavity and oropharynx for surgery of the mouth and is technically used for blind placement of the endotracheal tube more frequently than the orotracheal route. For the awake

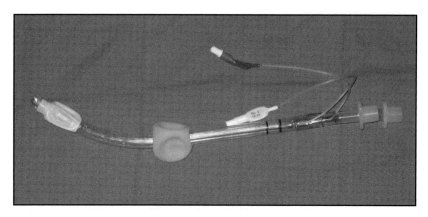

Fig 2–2. The Combitube™ has both a tracheal and an esophageal lumen as well as a pharyngeal cuff and a distal cuff to permit tracheal ventilation while minimizing the risk of aspiration.

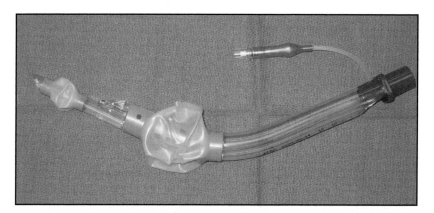

Fig 2–3. King Airway is a single lumen, dual cuff device that occludes the proximal oropharynx and obturates the distal end of the lumen in an attempt to occlude the esophageal lumen.

patient, the nasotracheal tube is better tolerated than the orotracheal tube. Similar to the orotracheal tube, the nasotracheal tube may be placed blindly, with the use of rigid or flexible laryngoscopes, or via a retrograde technique. If a standard laryngoscope is used to facilitate nasotracheal intubation, the tube is frequently guided into the larynx with special, nonpiercing forceps such as Magill or Rovenstine forceps. Nasotracheal tubes are not desirable as long-term airway solutions as these patients have a high risk of sinus infection and eustachian tube dysfunction.

Uncommonly, a submental approach to orotracheal intubation is used. It facilitates maxillomandibular fixation when nasotracheal intubation is not feasible such as when mid-face trauma and tracheostomy is undesirable. Submental intubation is facilitated by standard orotracheal intubation and confirming position standard techniques. Subsequently, an incision is made in the floor of the mouth lateral to the submandibular gland ducts and the attachments of the genioglossus muscle. The 15-mm endotracheal tube connector is removed and the endotracheal tube is placed through the incision to the outside neck and then the connector is replaced in proper position. The tube retains good tissue fixation and permits extubation after maxillomandibular fixation is placed and the patient is able to maintain their own airway. Preformed oral tubes such as the RAE™ tube or an armor tube are best suited for this clinical situation. They are less likely to kink and obstruct ventilation as opposed to standard orotracheal tubes.[8,9] If there are significant cosmetic considerations, the submental technique may create an unsightly scar.

AIDS TO INTUBATION

There are numerous devices and guides to facilitate endotracheal intubation. Examples of these include optical stylets, illuminating stylets for transtracheal visualization, and bougie-type stylets (Fig 2–4). In addition to the standard rigid laryngoscopes with their wide assortment of blade (Fig 2–5), there are flexible and rigid fiberoptic devices that permit direct visualization of the endotracheal tube as it passes over or through the device. Popular versions of the rigid devices include the Bullard Laryngoscope™, the Wu Scope™, and the Glide Scope™ (Fig 2–6).

As previously mentioned, there are uncommon but important techniques for intubation of the trachea. These include digital orotracheal intubation and

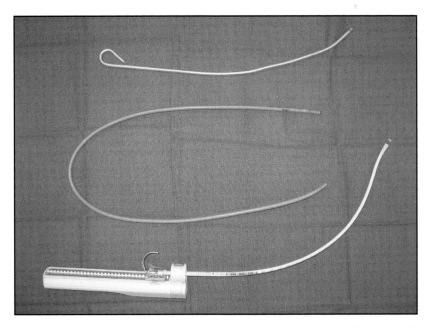

Fig 2–4. *Top*: Malleable Stylet, stays within tube; *Middle*: Gum-elastic bougie-extends beyond the tube (Eschmann Stylet); *Bottom*: Lighted stylet (Trach light).

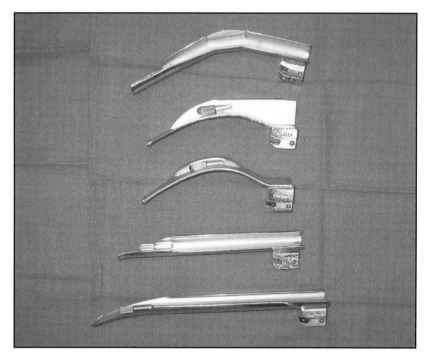

Fig 2–5. These are a wide assortment of rigid laryngoscope blades available.

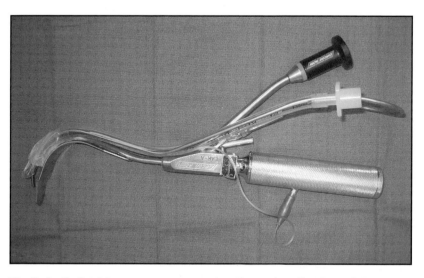

Fig 2–6. Bullard laryngoscope permits direct visualization of the endotracheal tube as it passes through the device.

retrograde orotracheal or nasotracheal intubation. The digital technique requires that the practitioner is able to palpate the epiglottis. Retrograde intubation requires that a large needle be placed through the cricothyroid membrane and a catheter or wire be passed into the oropharynx where it is tied to the Murphy eye of the endotracheal tube and then pulled into the trachea. These techniques require mannequin practice for the beginner. They are difficult to perform successfully under emergency circumstances without the mannequin practice. The pitfalls of the technique that may be encountered include detaching the catheter or anchor prior to completion of the procedure. Additionally, the tube may be malrotated in such a position as to prevent advancement through the larynx due to the edge of the tube catching on the arytenoids usually on the right side.

When the proximal airway is so severely obstructed as to prevent passage of any artificial airway, alternative methods of ventilation must be sought. High-frequency jet ventilation is a potential solution provided the jet ventilation catheter can be placed distal to the obstruction.[10] One such tube is a Benjamin tube. This tube has a small diameter, but, once in place, it moves very little in the distal trachea. The advantage of high-frequency jet ventilation is the low mean airway pressures in the face of rapid ventilation rates as high as 600 oscillations per minute. Unless there is total proximal obstruction to expired gas egress, normocapnia and acceptable oxygenation is maintained.

On rare occasions, the proximal subglottic airway is severely obstructed such that neither endotracheal intubation, catheter-mediated high-frequency jet ventilation, nor tracheotomies are satisfactory. In such a case, cardiopulmonary bypass initiated via the femoral route under local anesthesia may be necessary to assist in securing the airway. This technique is also known as extracorporeal membrane oxygenation (ECMO). A case in our experience involved a patient with almost complete midtracheal compression from a non-Hodgkin's lymphoma in the anterior mediastinum. The patient management team consisted of the oncologists, radiologists, otolaryngologists, anesthesiologists, and cardiothoracic surgeons. The patient was successfully managed in the previously described manner, the airway was secondarily secured with a rigid, ventilating bronchoscope after placement of femoral artery and femoral vein cannulae for bypass. Eventually, a tracheostomy was performed and a long tube was placed. The patient was discharged after external beam radiation on post-treatment day 10 with no known sequelae.[11] This technique has a significant risk of hemorrhage after heparinization for cardiopulmonary bypass. Therefore, the high risks and potential benefits must be weighed prior to this choice.[12]

Cricothyroidotomy with transtracheal ventilation is an invasive technique that places a ventilating needle or catheter through the cricothyroid membrane (Fig 2-7). It provides an alternative to tracheostomy for practitioners with minimal surgical experience. It is not meant to be a definitive airway. Its intent is to be a bridge to a more definitive airway such as an endotracheal tube or tracheostomy tube. Clinical situations that warrant such a device are the elective placement of such a catheter over a needle to facilitate ventilation during airway maneuvers or the only airway that is available on an emergent basis.[13] Ventilation through a cricothyroidotomy needle or catheter is usually limited by its narrow lumen. High-frequency jet ventilation is the most logical technique for this modality[14] (Fig 2-8). Once the transtracheal device is in place, it must be secured by the best means possible such as suture or by hand. The catheter is likely to be dislodged without definitive anchors during

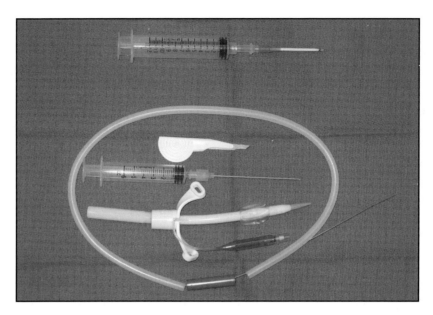

Fig 2–7. Cricothyroid device. *Top*: Simple needle and syringe; *Bottom*: Dilatational cricothyroidotomy kit.

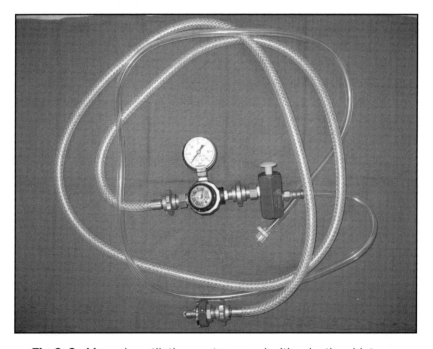

Fig 2–8. Manual ventilation system used with cricothyroidotomy.

any form of ventilation. There are many prepackaged kits that are specifically designed for cricothyroidotomy. How- ever, the simplest device consists of a 14-gauge IV catheter over a needle with an aspirating 10-cc syringe.

COMBINATIONS OF TECHNIQUES AND DEVICES

Clinical conditions develop such that no one technique or device will facilitate optimal patient outcome. A simple example of this problem is the patient that requires longer ventilation than anticipated during the initial assessment. Such a patient is transitioned from bag-mask-valve ventilation to orotracheal endotracheal intubation with continued ventilatory support. A more complex example of the combined techniques and devices may be necessary. In such a case, the Proseal™ laryngeal mask airway in conjunction with a distal position cricothyroidotomy device has been used successfully to manage the airway in a patient with both laryngeal and cricoid obstruction.[15] A summary of techniques and devices is presented in Tables 2–1 and 2–2.[16]

COMPLICATIONS OF ALTERNATIVES TO TRACHEOSTOMY

All techniques of airway management are associated with complications, many of which are minor and few of which are major. The prudent clinician should be aware of these complications prior to embarking upon the chosen approach.[17] Bag-valve-mask ventilation can result in insufflation of the stomach that may cause emesis and aspiration when airway pressures exceed 20 cm of water pressure. Twenty cm of water pressure is the threshold at which the gastroesophageal sphincter is opened by ventilation. If ventilation pressure is too high, the patient may also suffer barotrauma anywhere in the aerodigestive tract.

Table 2–1. Aids to Endotracheal Intubation

1. Intubating oropharyngeal airways
2. Semirigid solid stylets
3. Rigid solid bougie-type stylet guide
4. Hollow airway exchange catheter/ventilating stylets
5. Rigid optical stylets
6. Transilluminating light wands
7. Dental mirrors
8. Standard laryngoscopes
9. Prism laryngoscopes
10. Mirror laryngoscopes
11. Flexible fiberoptic laryngoscopes
12. Rigid fiberoptic laryngoscopes
13. Video laryngoscopes

Table 2–2. Techniques

1. Bag-valve-mask noninvasive technique
2. Bag-valve-mask with oropharyngeal or nasopharyngeal airway
3. Supraglottic ventilation with Laryngeal Mask Airway, Combitube, King Laryngeal Tube Device, or Cobra Perilaryngeal Tube
4. Subglottic ventilation with orotracheal, nasotracheal, or submental endotracheal tube
5. Cricothyroidotomy
6. Percutaneous wire-guided cricothyroidotomy
7. Combination of above techniques and devices
8. Cardiopulmonary bypass using femoral route (ECMO)

Bag-mask-valve manual ventilation may require the insertion of an oropharyngeal or nasopharyngeal airway to improve soft tissue obstruction. The tongue, the soft palate, and pharyngeal soft tissues may be stented by either type of airway. The oropharyngeal airway may worsen airway obstruction or cause soft tissue laceration if improperly placed. It also may be associated with dental trauma in the awake patient who is attempting to clench the teeth in a forceful manner. The nasopharyngeal airway is a soft and pliable device. However, it is associated with epistaxis and submucosal placement. It is unwise to place a nasopharyngeal airway in the presence of craniofacial trauma as there are sporadic reports of the airway lodging within a subarachnoid position.[18] It may also precipitate a latex allergy in the latex allergic patient if the red latex variety of tube is used.

Complications of endotracheal tube placement include complications similar to those of oropharyngeal and nasopharyngeal airway placement. Other complications are related directly to laryngoscopy including, trauma to the teeth, tongue, and temporomandibular joints including subluxation and dislocation. Placement of the nasotracheal tube is also associated with epistaxis, trauma to the turbinates, submucosal dissection, and possible inadvertent intracranial placement in the face of craniofacial trauma.[17,19]

All cuffed devices have several similar complications. All devices when overinflated are associated with local mucosal damage including the tracheal mucosa. In some instances, overinflation may be associated with occlusion of the main orifice of the airway. Such airway occlusion results in increased airway pressure and barotrauma if partially occluded and high risk of fatality if unrecognized in the complete occlusion.

Supralaryngeal devices may be associated with occasional pulmonary aspiration of gastric contents. The Cobra Perilaryngeal Airway™ has had one study stopped as a result of aspiration.[20] However, these devices may be life saving and the risk of pulmonary aspiration of gastric contents is preferable to the inevitable anoxic brain damage that would occur without these lifesaving devices. Aspiration pneumonia is frequently treatable and infrequently fatal. Anoxic brain damage is frequently fatal and rarely treatable.

All rigid devices are associated with mucosal damage and perforation; most of which are avoidable with the experienced clinician. Submucosal dissection caused by an endotracheal tube is more likely to occur in the blind passage of a nasotracheal tube than orotracheal tube. Submucosal dissection and subsequent attempts at manual or automated ventilation are commonly associated with submucosal emphysema that may dissect into the mediastinum, pericardium, or subcutaneous tissues.

Cricothyroidotomy is also associated with subcutaneous or submucosal emphysema if the needle or catheter device is not secured in place. Hemorrhage is rarely encountered if cricothyroidotomy is performed directly in the midline. However, in rapidly deteriorating situations, the midline of the neck may be missed and anterior venous structures may be entered.

SUMMARY

There are many alternative devices and techniques to tracheostomy in airway management. Each of these devices and techniques should be chosen based upon the clinical circumstances and practitioner experience with the alternatives. No one technique is applicable to all situations.

REFERENCES

1. Baillard C, Fosse JP, Sebbane M, et al. Noninvasive ventilation improves preoxygenation before intubation of hypoxic patients. *Am J Respir Crit Care Med.* 2006;174:71-177,

2. Esteban A, Frutos-Vivar F, Ferguson ND, et al. Noninvasive positive-pressure ventilation for respiratory failure after extubation. *N Engl J Med.* 2004;350: 2452-2460.

3. American Society of Anesthesiologists. Practice guidelines for management of the difficult airway: an updated report by the American Society of Anesthesiologists Task Force on management of the difficult airway. *Anesthesiology.* 2003;98: 1269-1277.

4. Ferson DZ, Rosenblatt WH, Johansen MJ. Use of the intubating LMA-Fastrach in 254 patients with difficult-to-manage airways. *Anesthesiology.* 2001;95:1175-1181.

5. McManus JG, Parson D, Prouix CA et al. Combat trauma airway management: Combitube™ versus the King laryngeal tracheal device by Army combat medic students. *Acad Emerg Med.* 2005;12 (suppl1):162.

6. Hagberg C, Bogomolny Y, Gilmore C, et al. An evaluation of the insertion and function of a new supraglottic airway device, the King LT™, during spontaneous ventilation. *Anesth Analg.* 2006; 102:621-625.

7. Gaitini L, Yanovski B, Somri M, et al. A comparison between the PLA Cobra™ and the Laryngeal Mask Airway Unique™ during spontaneous ventilation: a randomized prospective study. *Anesth Analg.* 2006;102:631-636.

8. Mahmood S, Lello GE. Oral endotracheal intubation: median submental (retroge-

nial) approach. *J Oral Maxillofac Surg.* 2002;60:474-475.

9. Arya VK, Kumar A, Makkar SS, et al. Retrograde submental intubation by pharyngeal loop technique in a patient with faciomaxillary trauma and restricted mouth opening. *Anesth Analg.* 2005; 100:534-537.

10. Alfille P. Anesthesia for tracheal surgery. In: Grillo HC. *Surgery of the Trachea and Bronchi.* Hamilton, Canada: BC Decker Inc; 2004:453-470

11. Petruzzelli GJ, deVries EJ, Johnson J, et al. Extrinsic tracheal compression from an anterior mediastinal mass in an adult: the multidisciplinary management of the airway emergency. *Otol Head Neck Surg.* 1990;103:484-486.

12. Grillo HC. Development of tracheal surgery: a historical review. In: Grillo HC. *Surgery of The Trachea and Bronchi.* Hamilton, Canada: BC Decker Inc; 2004:1-35.

13. Benumof JL, Scheller MS. The importance of transtracheal jet ventilation in the management of the difficult airway. *Anesthesiology.* 1989;71:769-778.

14. Klain M, Smith RB. High frequency percutaneous transtracheal ventilation. *Crit Care Med.* 1977;5:280-287.

15. Cook TM, Asif M, Sim R, et al. Use of a Proseal™ laryngeal mask airway and a Ravussin cricothyroidotomy needle in the management of laryngeal and subglottic stenosis causing upper airway obstruction. *Br J Anaesth.* 2005;95:554-557.

16. Orebaugh SL. *Atlas of Airway Management: Techniques and Tools.* Philadelphia, Pa: Lippincott Williams & Wilkins; 2007:75-209.

17. Herlich A. Complications from securing the difficult airway. *Int Anesth Clin.* 1997;35:13-30.

18. Muzzi DA, Losasso TJ, Cucchiara RF. Complications from a nasopharyngeal airway in a patient with a basilar skull fracture. *Anesthesiology.* 1991;74:366-368.

19. Hall CEJ, Shutt LE. Nasotracheal intubation for head and neck surgery. *Anaesthesia.* 2003;58:249-256.

20. Cook TM, Lowe JM. An evaluation of the Cobra Perilaryngeal Airway: study halted after two cases of pulmonary aspiration. *Anaesthesia.* 2005;60:791.

CHAPTER 3

Technique and Complications of Tracheostomy in Adults

ROHAN R. WALVEKAR
EUGENE N. MYERS

INTRODUCTION

Tracheostomy may be one of the easiest or one of the most difficult, dangerous, and frustrating of surgical procedures. When the procedure is elective, performed in the operating room on an adult with a slender neck and no airway obstruction, it is usually a simple, straightforward procedure attended by few if any problems. However, the procedure may be very difficult if the patient has a short, fat, or muscular neck, air hunger, or both. The number of risk factors increases when a tracheostomy is performed under less than ideal circumstances, as in the emergency department or at the bedside. Children requiring tracheostomy present special problems,

and the technique used to manage them must be modified in certain ways (see Chapter 4, "Technique and Complications of Tracheostomy in the Pediatric Age Group").

The highest priority before performing a tracheostomy is securing the airway. When performed electively in the patient without airway obstruction, as in a resection of a cancer of the head and neck, this is not usually a problem. If the patient has dyspnea from a compromised airway, an artificial airway may have to be inserted to ensure that the patient is well ventilated throughout the procedure. Endotracheal tubes are most often used today for securing the airway. In some circumstances, a rigid bronchoscope may be inserted, but few people in current practice are skilled in using this instrument, and this equipment is usually available only in the operating room. There are some patients who, because of a large obstructive laryngeal tumor, cervical trauma, or anatomic abnormality will not be able to be intubated and will have an emergency tracheostomy under local anesthesia. This will provide an airway that may need to be modified once the emergency has been relieved and the patient stabilized.

Tracheostomy is most safely and easily performed in the operating room, where adequate light, suction, and assistants are available. Patients who have arrived in the emergency department with an endotracheal tube in place or who are intubated in the emergency department[1] should be transferred to the operating room for this procedure despite the cost. Hospitalized patients, particularly those in an intensive care unit, usually have the tracheostomy performed at the bedside.

INDICATIONS FOR TRACHEOSTOMY

There are numerous indications for tracheostomy. Some of the more commonly encountered indications are listed below:

- Airway obstruction due to an:
  - Abnormality outside the tracheal lumen (eg, compressive thyroid mass, anomaly of the great vessels)
  - Abnormality within the tracheal lumen (eg, primary tracheal tumor)
  - Abnormality within the tracheal wall (eg, severe tracheomalacia)
  - Abnormalities of the supraglottis or glottis (eg, congenital anomalies, stenosis, infection, tumor, bilateral vocal cord paralysis)
- Trauma to the neck that causes severe injury to the laryngeal framework, great vessels, or the hyoid bone.
- Subcutaneous emphysema
- Comminuted fractures of the midface and mandible (traumatic or iatrogenic as a part of orthognathic surgery)
- Edema of the airway due to trauma, burns, infection, or anaphylaxis
- For patients requiring long-term ventillatory support (eg, comatose patients, patients with respiratory failure)
- To provide access for adequate pulmonary toilet especially in patients with chronic aspiration and those who are unable to cough due to chronic pain or weakness
- Elective airway management in conjunction with extensive head and neck oncologic resections and/or brachytherapy for head neck cancers
- Obstructive sleep apnea.

PERIOPERATIVE MANAGEMENT

Position of Patient

The patient is placed on the operating table or other firm surface with a rolled towel or sheet under the shoulders to extend the neck (Fig 3–1). This brings the trachea more anterior in the neck and exposes more of its length. A small pillow or rubber "doughnut" should be placed

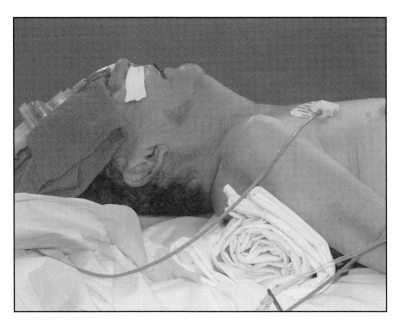

Fig 3-1. Positioning of patient for tracheostomy with a rolled blanket under the shoulder to extend the head.

under the patient's head to stabilize it during surgery. Some patients with obstruction of the airway cannot tolerate lying supine, and in these patients the tracheostomy must be performed under local anesthesia with the patient in a sitting or semisitting position. In other patients, such as those with cervical osteoarthritis, questionable or documented fractures of the cervical spine, or severe kyphoscoliosis, the neck cannot be extended.

Anesthesia

Tracheostomy in adults may be carried out under local or general anesthesia. In patients with a difficult airway, use of a local anesthetic allows spontaneous respiration until the airway is secured. General anesthesia can be induced, if needed, once the tracheostomy has provided a secure airway. Many patients

requiring tracheostomy are at high risk of respiratory distress either because of existing airway obstruction or because of associated medical or surgical problems. When possible, these patients should undergo oral or nasal endotracheal intubation before tracheostomy to secure the airway and to prevent struggling during the procedure. Patients from the intensive care unit who are being maintained by mechanical ventilation or bagging through an endotracheal tube may also undergo a tracheostomy under local anesthesia.

The line of incision should be marked on the skin prior to placing the patient in extension and before the local anesthesia is injected. Whenever possible the incision for the tracheostomy should be incorporated into the incision for the neck dissection. When using local anesthesia, Xylocaine 1% with 1:100,000 epinephrine should be injected into the skin and subcutaneous tissue where the incision for the tracheostomy has been outlined. Although the anesthetic takes effect instantly after injection, it takes approximately 5 to 10 minutes for the vasoconstrictive effect of the epinephrine to develop. In nonemergency situations, the local anesthetic is injected and while the vasoconstriction is developing the patient can be prepared and draped for surgery. In patients undergoing tracheostomy under general anesthesia, it is not necessary to inject local anesthesia. Hemostasis can be secured with electrocautery or sutures.

Preparation of the Patient

After the airway has been secured and the patient has been positioned correctly, the face, neck, chest, and shoulder should be sterilized with prep solution and the patient draped to allow easy access to the neck. We do not drape the face. Patients who have not been intubated may receive oxygen by nasal catheter. This catheter should be either prepared with antiseptic solution or draped out of the operative field. When electrocautery is used, the anesthetist must be notified prior to the use of cautery to stop the flow of oxygen to prevent an explosion or a fire.

SURGICAL TECHNIQUE

Creation of the Stoma

A transverse incision is made in the skin approximately 1 cm above the suprasternal notch, in the triangle (Jackson's triangle) bounded by the cricoid cartilage superiorly and the medial aspect of the sternocleidomastoid muscles (Fig 3–2). Sharp dissection is carried down

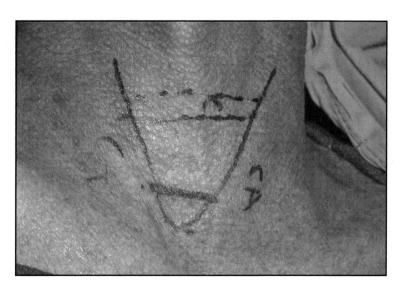

Fig 3-2. Jackson's triangle with solid lines indicating the anterior border of the sternocleidomastoid muscles with position of carotid arteries (*CA*) lateral and the cricoid cartilage superiorly with dotted and solid lines.

through the subcutaneous tissue. The rake side of a pair of Senn retractors is used to retract the superior and inferior skin flap. Using the blunt side the anterior jugular veins are identified and retracted (Fig 3-3A). The strap muscles are separated in the midline and retracted laterally (Fig 3-3B). The thyroid isthmus is visualized and the anterior wall of the trachea is identified.

The isthmus of the thyroid is retracted superiorly with the rake end of the Senn retractor. In most cases, it is not necessary to transect the isthmus of the thyroid. Should transection of the isthmus be necessary, it is done most easily by undermining the isthmus and placing right-angle clamps on each side of the isthmus. The isthmus is then transected and the cut edges of the isthmus oversewn with silk sutures to prevent bleeding. Some surgeons prefer to transect the isthmus using electrocautery without using sutures. Proper retraction of the strap muscles and the thyroid isthmus will provide excellent exposure of the trachea. If the dissection is kept in the midline there should be a bloodless field.

Once the trachea had been exposed in the awake patient, a small amount of local anesthesia is infiltrated into the anterior wall of the trachea to eliminate pain (see Fig 3-3B). It is important to limit dissection to the anterior wall of the trachea in order to prevent pneumothorax, pneumomediastinum, or subcutaneous emphysema.

It is important to palpate the cricoid cartilage to determine the level at which to enter the trachea. In the patient with a cuffed endotracheal tube in place it may be prudent, to avoid puncturing the cuff, to have the cuff deflated prior to making the incision in the trachea. An incision is made in the interspace between the second and third tracheal rings. Once this incision is made, a

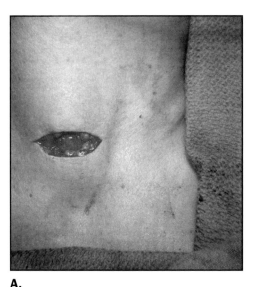
A.

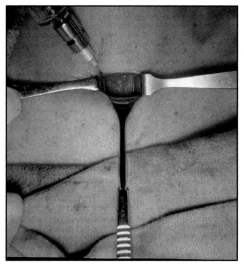
B.

Fig 3-3. A. Good visualization of the anterior jugular veins. **B.** Medial edge of strap muscles visualized, retracted, and the trachea skeletonized. Local anesthesia injected into the peritracheal tissues.

tracheal hook should be placed so that it engages the tracheal ring above the incision from within the trachea. Another transverse incision is then made below the third tracheal ring. In older patients, the tracheal ring is calcified and may not be cut with a scalpel, so a heavy curved Mayo scissor can be used to cut vertically through the tracheal ring on the side closest to the surgeon. The cut edge of the tracheal ring is then grasped with an Allis clamp and cut through on the far side (Fig 3–4A), leaving a window in the trachea. It is important to grasp the cartilage ring firmly to prevent it from falling into or being aspirated into the tracheobronchial tree. If necessary, the stoma may then be enlarged by removing additional cartilage laterally with a Kerrison rongeur. Removal of the anterior aspect of the tracheal ring ensures that the tracheostomy tube is placed in the trachea rather than in a false passage anterior to the trachea. It also provides a comfortable and secure fit of the cannula in the trachea and provides an ample opening for future changes of the tracheostomy tube.

Traction Sutures

Traction sutures are used to facilitate reinsertion of the tracheostomy cannula in the event it should become dislodged in the immediate postoperative period before a tract has formed.[2] We recommend 2-0 silk sutures. A ligature passer is often easier to manipulate in the depths of the wound than a curved needle (Fig 3–4B). While the tracheal hook retracts the superior aspect of the trachea inferiorly into the wound, the ligature passer is passed through the interspace just above the ring superior to the stoma and

into the lumen, care being taken not to penetrate the posterior wall of the trachea. A small curved clamp is used to grasp the suture while the ligature passer is removed. A similar procedure is carried out in the ring inferior to the stoma. Once the sutures are placed, traction is applied to both sutures to exteriorize the tracheal stoma and retract the skin edges (Fig 3–4C). At this time, either a tracheostomy tube or an endotracheal tube is inserted, according to the patient's needs.

The traction sutures provide an extra measure of safety in the immediate postoperative period. If the tracheostomy tube is accidentally dislodged, it may be difficult or impossible to replace as a tract from the skin to the trachea has not yet formed. If the tracheostomy tube that has been dislodged is forced into the newly formed stoma a false passage between the anterior wall of the trachea and the sternum may be created in which case the patient's airway is severely compromised. This is true in the nursing unit that does not have sufficient light or proper instruments, particularly in a restless, uncooperative patient with airway obstruction. If the patient has had traction sutures placed, the airway can be exteriorized by pulling up on the traction sutures and then holding them parallel to the chest. This maneuver retracts the skin edges and pulls the stoma into the wound, thereby re-establishing the airway until such time that the tracheostomy tube or an endotracheal tube can be inserted.

Cannulation

Once the traction sutures have been satisfactorily placed, the tracheostomy tube is

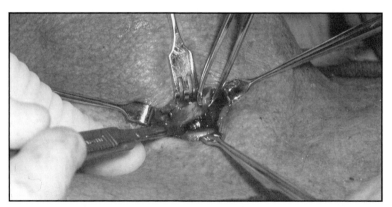

A.

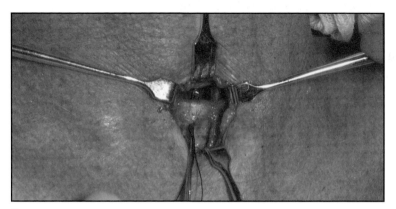

B.

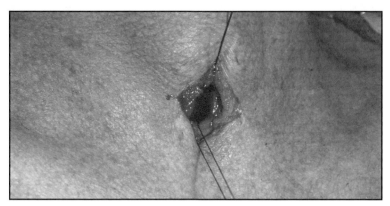

C.

Fig 3-4. A. The trachea is entered through an incision between the second and third tracheal rings as the thyroid isthmus is retracted superiorly. The tracheal ring is grasped with an Allis clamp and a portion of the tracheal ring is removed to form a window in the trachea **B.** A ligature passer is used to place a traction suture through the space below the tracheal ring. **C.** Traction sutures are placed superior and inferior to the stoma in adults.

inserted into the stoma (Fig 3-5). This is begun with the tube at right angles to the trachea; then, as the tube is inserted, it is rotated so that its axis is parallel to that of the trachea. This eliminates the difficulty encountered in trying to pass the cannula over the patient's chest at a difficult angle to the stoma. For ease and

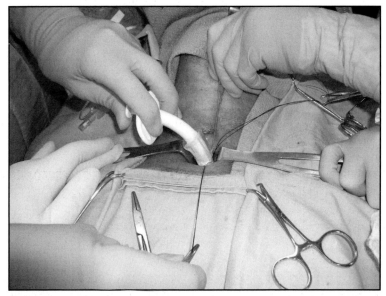

A.

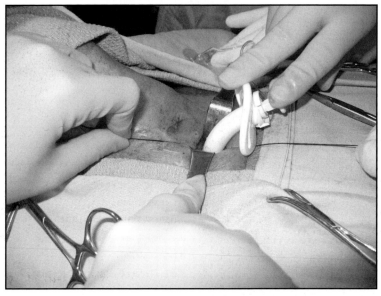

B.

Fig 3-5. A. The tracheostomy tube is inserted into the trachea initially from the side. **B.** The tracheostomy tube is then rotated into the trachea and the obturator removed.

accuracy of insertion an obturator should always be used when the tube is being inserted. Once the tube is properly seated in the trachea, the obturator is removed promptly and the inner cannula inserted. If an endotracheal tube or bronchoscope had been used to stabilize the airway, it must be removed from the area of the stoma but it should not be removed entirely until the tracheostomy tube is securely in place. The neck plate of the tracheostomy tube has two slots originally designed to accommodate the umbilical tape (twill) used to hold the tube in place. We use 2-0 silk sutures (Fig 3-6) inserted through these slots to sew the neck plate to the skin. This is a great safety feature to prevent accidental dislodgement of the tracheostomy tube in the early postoperative period.

In cases in which the tracheostomy is performed preoperatively for postoperative management of the airway an endotracheal tube is inserted when the tracheostomy is established. At the end of the procedure when the patient is breathing spontaneously, the endotracheal tube is removed and the tracheostomy tube is inserted by bringing the trachea into the wound with the traction sutures. Right-angle retractors are then used to provide adequate exposure and the tube is inserted accurately and sutured to the skin as described above.

At the time of the initial tube change which takes place (on average) on the sixth postoperative day the sutures are removed and a Velcro neck strap is applied to keep the tracheostomy tube in place. The tube change is done by the surgeons. In most hospitals nonphysicians are not allowed to make the first tracheostomy tube change (nurses do, however, change the inner cannula). It is mandatory that adequate light, suction, and assistance are available. In patients undergoing total laryngectomy, the sutures are not necessary except in patients with pectoralis flap reconstruction or patients with a low cervical incision for neck dissections

TRACHEOSTOMY: CREATION OF A PERMANENT STOMA

After the tracheostomy is performed a tract forms around the tube. Granulation tissue develops in the tract and the tract is difficult to keep clean. When a permanent tract or tracheostomy is desired, the surgical technique should be modified somewhat to facilitate early healing and maintenance of hygiene. This is especially important when frequent access to the trachea is necessary, as in patients with permanent laryngeal stenosis, severe chronic obstructive lung disease, sleep apnea, or those who will be permanently ventilator-dependent. Permanent epithelialization of the tracheostomy is

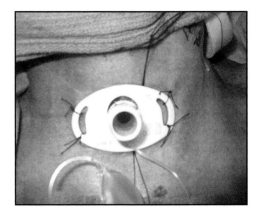

Fig 3-6. The neck plate of the tracheostomy tube is sutured to the skin to avoid the use of tapes.

facilitated when a skin-to-mucosa tract is created at the initial surgery. A number of complex skin flap procedures have been described, but we feel that these are, generally, unnecessary. Furthermore, complete circumferential skin-to-mucosa closure has frequently resulted in the development of wound infection, with disruption of the suture line and the formation of difficult-to-manage granulation tissue.

We try to establish a skin-to-mucosa tract by making a horizontal skin incision 1 cm inferior to the cricoid cartilage. The incision is carried down to the level of the strap muscles. Skin flaps are then elevated approximately 2 cm, both superiorly and inferiorly. The subcutaneous adipose tissue is then removed. The amount of soft tissue removed depends in large part on the reason for the permanent tracheostomy and the patient's body habitus. Frequently, large amounts of adipose tissue are removed from obese patients who are having a permanent tracheostomy to treat sleep apnea (see Chapter 8 "Tracheostomy in Patients with Obstructive Sleep Apnea Syndrome").

The strap muscles are then separated in the midline and retracted laterally. The thyroid isthmus will be encountered and should be divided in the midline and oversewn. The thyroid is then retracted laterally to expose the trachea. An inferiorly based tracheal flap is then made with either the second and third or third and fourth tracheal rings. The tracheal flap is rotated inferiorly and sutured to the skin flap. Redundant skin should be trimmed. The superior skin flap is brought down and sutured to the superior aspect of the tracheal wall. No attempt should be made to close the triangular lateral defects, which will heal by secondary intention. The patient is maintained with a tracheostomy tube or button, as the case may indicate. This technique facilitates rapid healing and the establishment of an epithelial tract.

POSTOPERATIVE CARE AND AN ALGORITHM FOR DECANNULATION

Postoperative care is critical. The introduction of the tracheostomy tube stimulates the trachea to produce copious secretions. In the immediate postoperative period, we suggest regular suctioning of the tracheal secretions with simultaneous irrigation using sterile saline available in prepackaged saline bullets. Tracheal suctioning is performed as often as half-hourly and then titrated to suit the patient's needs. It is vital that tracheal suctioning should be performed gently and the suction tubing not be inserted beyond the length of the tube to prevent tracheal ulceration and tracheitis. Humidified oxygen helps to prevent drying and inspissation of mucous secretions and also prevents air drying the tracheal mucosa. The inner cannula of the tracheostomy tube should be removed and cleaned at least twice daily. This avoids the accumulation of dried mucus from forming plugs which may occlude the inner cannula, a potentially life-threatening situation. When a cuffed tracheostomy tube is inserted, it is ideal to deflate the cuff periodically as indicated to avoid pressure necrosis of the tracheal mucosa. Excessive traction on the tracheostomy tube should be prevented by providing adequate support and stabilization of the tube; this is especially true for patients who are on ventillatory support and have heavy tubing connecting the tracheostomy tube to the ventilator.

The nurses may remove, clean, or change the inner cannula, but not the tracheostomy tube itself. The first complete tube change is done (on average) on the sixth postoperative day. The tube change is accomplished at the bedside by the physician. This is potentially dangerous if fibrosis between the tracheostoma and skin has not formed. It is mandatory to have present: adequate light (preferably a head-light), suction, instruments, and experienced assistants. The patient's head should be positioned in extension similar to the position used when the tracheostomy was performed. This "lines up" the skin incision with the trachostoma. Patient education as well as education of the patient's caregivers with respect to the care of the tracheostomy tube should be started as soon as possible. This is more pertinent to patients who will need to have the tracheostomy tube for prolonged periods of time.

The tube change is performed by the physician by first cutting out the silk sutures that have been placed at the time of insertion of the tracheostomy tube to secure the neck plate to the skin. The tracheostomy tube is then removed and the stoma occluded by the surgeon's thumb to test the patient's ability to breathe and speak through their normal airway. If the patient does not have a sufficient airway, then the No. 6 cuffed Shiley tube is replaced as these patients still are at high risk for losing their airway should the tube become dislodged, with the ever present danger of death as a consequence. Over the next several days, the patient's airway is then tested each day and when it appears satisfactory, then downsizing may proceed. Our usual method of managing the decannulation

process of the patient who has had a major head and neck procedure with a tracheostomy tube is as follows: As it usually takes 5 to 6 days for the patient to regain the ability to swallow and for the laryngeal edema to subside, we usually do not make any earlier changes to the tracheostomy tube. On average, about the sixth postoperative day, the cuff is deflated and the patient's ability to tolerate the secretions and test the patency of the airway by occluding the tube is carried out. In an adult, a No. 6 Shiley tube with the cuff deflated leaves enough room in the trachea for the patient to breathe around the tube. If the patient demonstrates that they can speak and breathe through the mouth, then we feel that downsizing is appropriate.

If the patient does do well with the tube occluded, then a No. 4 uncuffed Shiley tube is inserted. Once downsized, a Passey-Muir valve may be placed on the inner cannula which allows the patient to speak and improves swallowing function as well. If the patient does well with the No. 4 uncuffed Shiley tube, the tube is removed over the next several days and the stoma occluded. If the patient does tolerate occlusion of the airway, then the tracheostomy tube is removed and a dressing of gauze and tape is secured in place over the stoma. Finger occlusion of this dressing creates a better seal around the stoma to help the patient speak and swallow.

Some patients will not be able to be decannulated in the early postoperative period following the tracheostomy. They will be discharged with their tracheostomy tube in place. If the patient is going home the spouse or other caregiver must be instructed about the care of the tracheostomy. If the patient is to be discharged to a skilled nursing facility, proper communication with the nurses at the facility should be instituted (see Chapter 9 on Nursing Care). The patient will be evaluated in the surgeons office and decannulation arranged at the appropriate time.

COMPLICATIONS OF TRACHEOSTOMY

Even with the use of optimal surgical techniques, complications of tracheostomy may occur during the procedure, in the immediate postoperative period, or long after surgery. The best way of preventing complications is by paying meticulous attention to detail and by performing the tracheostomy as soon as it becomes obvious that the procedure is necessary. The complications of tracheostomy in adults are reviewed, and the means to prevent or manage each of them is discussed.

Intraoperative Complications

Hemorrhage

Prevention. When possible, a careful history is sought regarding coagulation disorders, such as may occur in patients with liver disease, hemophilia, leukemia, and coagulopathies or other hematologic disorders. Screening with formal coagulation studies and consultation with a hematologist are indicated in such patients when possible prior to the tracheostomy. The use of medications such as anticoagulants, aspirin, and non-steroidal anti-inflammatory drugs may contribute to excess bleeding during the procedure as well as in the immediate

postoperative period. Unfortunately this information may not be available in an unconscious patient or in an emergency situation.

Bleeding during the procedure has been categorized as unusual, excessive, major, and massive bleeding. Unusual bleeding is any amount of bleeding considered "abnormal" by the person performing the procedure. Excessive bleeding is more than 20 mL of estimated blood loss. Major bleeding is defined as a decrease in the hematocrit of ≥ 3 points, or transfusion of ≥ 2 units of packed red cells. Massive bleeding is considered to be a decrease in the hematocrit of ≥ 6 points, or transfusion of ≥ 2 units of packed red cells.[3] The frequency of major and minor bleeding for tracheostomy has been reported to occur in 0 to 7% and 0 to 80% of procedures, respectively.[4]

Bleeding during the performance of a tracheostomy may be prevented or minimized by meticulous attention to the details of the procedure. The patient's airway should be secure and the patient restrained, if necessary, to eliminate the possibility that the patient might disrupt the procedure by spontaneous movements. If the tracheostomy is to be performed under a local anesthetic, the procedure should not begin until the vasoconstriction produced by the local infiltration is complete. This helps immensely to prevent intra and postoperative oozing.

During the procedure, structures such as the anterior jugular veins and the thyroid isthmus must be identified carefully so that they will not be transected inadvertently. Although some capillary oozing is to be expected, the wound must otherwise be dry before the tracheostomy tube is inserted. In particular, dissection should be confined to the midline and all surgical landmarks must be identified to avoid lacerating the carotid artery. Such an occurrence may be prevented by ensuring that the procedure is kept under control at all times and that adequate lighting, equipment, and personnel are available.

Any peristomal bleeding should be thoroughly investigated. Hemorrhage occurring within the first 48 hours is typically associated with local factors such as injury to the anterior jugular veins, inferior thyroid veins, systemic coagulopathy, and tracheal erosions secondary to excessive suctioning or bronchopneumonia. Another vascular structure that may be at risk is an aberrant innominate artery.[5] If the stoma is placed low on the trachea, this vessel may be seen overlying the trachea (Fig 3-7), in the anterior superior mediastinum, and it should be recognized and protected. Pulsation of the tracheostomy tube once inserted may be a sign that the tube is pressing on the innominate artery; if possible, the tracheostomy site should be changed.

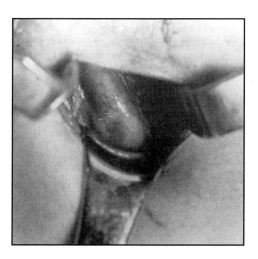

Fig 3-7. Innominate artery lying on the anterior wall of the trachea

Treatment. Once the tracheostomy tube has been inserted, the patient should be observed so that any bleeding problems resulting directly from the surgery may be identified. Bleeding may become apparent when a patient who has been hypotensive re-establishes normal blood pressure. In such cases the source of bleeding must be identified. In other cases introduction of the tracheostomy tube may cause a paroxysm of coughing and vessels in the skin around the stoma may bleed and require cautery.

If persistent bleeding occurs from a site deep in the wound, the tracheostomy tube must be removed and deep retractors and suction used to identify and ligate the bleeding vessels. If the surgeon merely packs the wound tightly with gauze to prevent bleeding, the patient may develop subcutaneous emphysema. In most cases, minor bleeding can be controlled by electrocautery or suture ligation.

Intraoperative Tracheoesophageal Fistula (TEF)

To avoid creating a fistula between the posterior wall of the trachea and the anterior wall of the esophagus, the surgeon must be careful not to penetrate the posterior wall of the trachea. Opening the trachea over a bronchoscope or endotracheal tube and then enlarging the incision will help to avoid injuring the trachea. This reiterates the importance of performing a tracheostomy in a controlled environment in the operating room with endotracheal intubation whenever possible. When the traction sutures are inserted, the ligature passer should be introduced at a shallow angle to the trachea so that the posterior wall of the trachea is not punctured. Removing a portion of the cartilaginous ring and adequate light will allow visualization of this area and help to avoid this complication. Identification of the trachea correctly prior to making an incision is vital and helps to prevent such iatrogenic injuries. The trachea can be difficult to locate in certain situations such as previous neck surgery, neck masses, obesity, short stature (bull neck), cervical arthritis, and kyphoscoliosis. In these situations identification of the trachea can be facilitated by the use of a tracheostomy guide, fiberoptic bronchoscope, or the use of Trachlight (originally developed to facilitate light-guided intubation techniques).[6] Finally, the posterior tracheal wall should be inspected just before insertion of the tracheostomy tube to confirm that the wall is intact.

If the tracheal wall has been injured and a fistula created, it should be repaired immediately. After the neck has been opened, the trachea should be dissected away from the esophagus and each structure repaired separately. Soft tissues such as a flap from the strap or sternocleidomastoid muscles should be interposed between the suture lines of the esophagus and trachea so that the risk of recurrence of the fistula is decreased. Before the wound is closed, a drain should be inserted in the neck; perioperative antibiotics should be administered; and, postoperatively, the patient should be fed through a nasogastric tube until the fistula is completely healed. TEF also can as a delayed complication of tracheostomy as a result of tracheostomy cuff injury, erosion from a plastic nasogastric tube, or direct injury.[7] Antibiotics should be administered to prevent infection in this contaminated area.

Pneumothorax

Pneumothorax occurs infrequently in adults undergoing tracheostomy, but when it does occur, it is usually the result of the rupture of a pulmonary bleb as a patient suffering from air hunger struggles to breath. This also can result from direct injury to the pleura by the surgeon. It occurs more often in children because the pleural dome protrudes into the lower neck and thus is more vulnerable to injury. In fact, one of the most frequently occurring complications associated with tracheostomy in the pediatric age group is the development of interstitial air (emphysema, pneumomediastinum, and pneumothorax). Pneumothorax occurs in up to 17% of children older than 12 months, in up to 4% of infants, and in up to 28% of premature babies or newborns.[8] Pneumothorax can also result from inadvertent damage to the posterior tracheal wall and esophagus as a result of knife contact or excessive force during tube insertion. Treatment includes evaluation of the posterior wall of the trachea by direct inspection and closure of the laceration through the tracheostomy stoma.[9]

Pneumothorax may also occur when the tracheostomy tube is inserted between the anterior wall of the trachea and the soft tissues of the anterior mediastinum, creating a false passage (Fig 3–8).[10] This condition is diagnosed when the patient does not have an adequate airway after intubation. If positive pressure breathing is initiated while the tube is lodged in the soft tissues of the neck marked subcutaneous emphysema, pneumomediastinum, and pneumothorax will result. False passage must be considered in the differential diagnosis of worsening respiratory status after

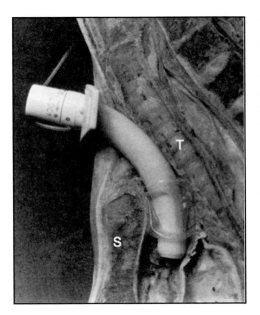

Fig 3-8. Sagittal section through the neck and chest of a cadaver, demonstrating a false passage of the tracheostomy tube between the sternum and the trachea (*T* = trachea, *S* = sternum).

insertion of the tracheostomy tube. Inability to insert a suction catheter through the tracheostomy tube into the trachea is also a clue as to the nature of this complication. All patients should be evaluated radiographically after the tracheostomy tube has been inserted to verify that it is in the correct position and to rule out pneumothorax.

Pneumothorax is best prevented by establishing an airway before tracheostomy is begun and by making sure that the stoma is made at the correct level on the trachea. The tracheostomy should be inserted under direct observation with good illumination and the patient, if awake and breathing spontaneously, should be directed to breathe deeply as the surgeon feels the flow of air through the tube; if the patient is under general anesthesia, the position of

the tube should be checked by inserting a suction catheter. It is important to communicate with the anesthesiologist to be certain that end tidal CO_2 is present to confirm intubation of the airway. If the patient is to be ventilated mechanically through the tube, this should be attempted cautiously while the endotracheal tube or bronchoscope is still in place. If any doubt remains as to whether the tube is located in the trachea, retractors should be placed in the stoma to keep it open, and the tube should be removed and placed into the trachea under direct vision. If the stoma is too low on the trachea for the tracheostomy tube to be inserted, a new stoma must be created superiorly. Injury to the posterior wall of the trachea and resulting pneumothorax can be avoided by use of a properly executed tracheostomy and careful insertion of the tube.[9] When pneumothorax is symptomatic, it should be treated by inserting a chest tube.

Pneumomediastinum

Asymptomatic pneumomediastinum occurs frequently in children and is discovered on routine chest radiographs. When pneumomediastinum does occur, its treatment depends upon the amount of air present. A small amount of air usually will be absorbed without difficulty, but when a large volume of air is present and/or the patient is symptomatic, it may be necessary to insert chest tubes to relieve the condition. This complication also may arise when patients struggling to breathe against obstruction pull air into the mediastinum. To avoid this complication an airway always should be established before the procedure is begun. Another cause of pneumomediastinum is excessive coughing, which forces air from the open tracheostomy into the deeper planes of the neck.

Pneumomediastinum is one of the most frequently encountered consequences of tracheostomy and is usually noted on the chest radiograph. In children older than 12 months it occurs in up to 43% of cases, whereas it occurs in up to 28% of children under 12 months.[8] The development of this problem seems to be related to the extent of peritracheal dissection during the procedure.[11] The surgeon should be aware of this technical feature and limit the dissection to the anterior wall of the trachea.

Injury to the Recurrent Laryngeal Nerve

The recurrent laryngeal nerve lies in the tracheoesophageal sulcus and should never be injured during tracheostomy if the dissection is limited to the midline. Because this nerve innervates the vocal cord, it is not possible to evaluate its integrity in the patient with a tracheostomy other than by direct or flexible laryngoscopy; if the nerve has been injured, laryngoscopy will reveal paralysis of the vocal cord.

If it is certain that the recurrent laryngeal nerve has been cut during tracheostomy, an intraoperative vocal cord medialization procedure may be carried out to fix the vocal cord in the midline or a decision may be made to observe the patient and, if necessary, carry out a secondary procedure. However, if injury is suspected but not certain, the patient should be re-examined at intervals for at least 6 months postoperatively to monitor return of vocal cord function. If there has been no improvement in this period of time, it is unlikely that recovery will occur spontaneously.[12]

When the extent of injury to the recurrent nerve is unclear and the patient has symptoms and endoscopic findings of recurrent laryngeal nerve dysfunction (weak voice with or without aspiration), Gelfoam has been used successfully in providing temporary medialization of the vocal cord without any adverse effects.[13] The judgment as to which patient needs Gelfoam injection depends on the degree of aspiration, the patient's general condition, and their own personal needs. A material has been developed recently for the treatment of temporary vocal cord paresis/palsy of uncertain permanency. It is made of gelatin, carboxymethycellulose, and water and is a good alternative to Gelfoam. It satisfies several properties of the ideal temporary vocal fold injection material such as effectiveness, biocompatibility, easy availability, ease of use and administration, reduced resorbtion rate that makes it effective for several months, and ability to simulate the bioelastic properties of the vocal cord.[13] However, if the patient does not regain function of the vocal cord in 6 months a thyroplasty/medialization procedure should be performed to rehabilitate the voice.

In the event of bilateral recurrent laryngeal nerve injury during tracheostomy, the patient will have airway difficulties and a breathy voice, which will become evident when decannulation is attempted. If such patients do not recover function spontaneously in 6 months, a medial arytenoidectomy or a transverse cordotomy are both good options to increase the glottic airway.[14]

Cricoid Cartilage Injury

Before Chevalier Jackson alerted surgeons not to violate the cricoid cartilage in performing a tracheostomy,[15] this structure was frequently injured, resulting in chondritis with subsequent formation of subglottic stenosis. If the cricoid cartilage is inadvertently injured during the tracheostomy, the tube should be removed and a new stoma created in a location more inferior on the trachea. The patients seen with subglottic stenosis have often been subject to an emergency tracheostomy, often done by someone not an expert in this field, who violates inadvertently this important landmark. Various techniques to treat subglottic stenosis are available.

Cardiopulmonary Arrest

Etiology. Although tracheostomy is considered a life-saving procedure, it may also lead to life-threatening complications. Cardiopulmonary arrest may result if the tube is placed improperly, as into a false passage; pulmonary edema occurs; or the tracheostomy is performed too low on the trachea and the lumen of the tube is occluded by the anterior wall of the trachea. Pneumomediastinum and tension pneumothorax caused by positive pressure ventilation also may lead to cardiopulmonary arrest.

Paradoxically, respiratory arrest followed by cardiac arrest may occur on opening the trachea of a patient who has chronic upper respiratory obstruction. The mechanism is thought to be the result of sudden loss of the hypoxemic stimulus to the chemoreceptor centers, which had been depressed by the constantly elevated levels of CO_2. The hypoxemia and acidosis that occur accentuate myocardial irritability and may precipitate cardiac arrest.[16]

Sudden relief of airway obstruction can result in the sudden onset of pulmonary edema. The mechanism of development is multifactorial and seems to be related to hypoxia, profound hemodynamic changes occurring during respiration, and possibly the disruption of the pulmonary endothelium. The hemodynamics of the inspiratory and expiratory phase of respiration are disrupted by introduction of the tracheostomy tube, resulting in an increase in systemic venous return and with resultant pulmonary edema.[17]

Prevention. When a patient suffering from chronic upper respiratory tract obstruction is to undergo a tracheostomy, the procedure should be performed with an anesthesiologist in attendance to monitor the patient. The anesthesiologist should be alerted that respiratory arrest may occur. A cuffed endotracheal tube must be readily available to insert into the trachea to facilitate resuscitation and increase the patient's oxygenation until hypoxemia has been overcome and the patient's central chemoreceptor response has been re-established.

When the patient develops sudden pulmonary edema upon insertion of the tracheostomy tube, continuous positive airway pressure (CPAP) ventilation must be instituted. Such patients should be cared for in an intensive care unit. The application of moderate CPAP in conjunction with administration of diuretics usually clears the pulmonary edema within 24 hours, and also prevents the onset of pulmonary edema when acute obstruction is relieved.[18] Although this type of pulmonary edema can be seen after severe and prolonged obstruction, it is often misdiagnosed or may go unrecognized.[17] Hence, it is important for the physician to be aware of this complication and always keep a high index of suspicion to be able to diagnose and treat this complication effectively.

Complications in the Immediate Postoperative Period

Postoperative Hemorrhage

Bleeding may occur in the early postoperative period when the vasoconstrictive effect of the epinephrine in the anesthetic solution wears off. Although such bleeding may be coming from vessels that were lacerated during surgery and not repaired, prolonged oozing should make the surgeon suspect a coagulation defect.

If only a small amount of blood is oozing from the wound and the patient has a cuffed tracheostomy tube, the wound may be packed lightly; but if bleeding is brisk, the patient must be taken back to the operating room, the wound explored, and hemostasis achieved either with electrocautery or suture ligation.

Wound Infection

The area around a tracheostomy is quickly colonized by many species of organisms, including most commonly *Pseudomonas* and *Escherichia coli* as well as gram-positive organisms. However, there is usually no sign of infection around the stoma, and if an infection becomes evident, it usually responds well to local treatment.

Nevertheless, serious wound infections may occur. After tracheostomy, wound care is important to decrease abnormal granulation and subcutaneous abscesses.[19] Necrotizing infections of the tracheostomy site have been described which can result in loss of tracheal tissue, large air leaks, and life-threatening hemorrhage.[20] Patients with a long-term tracheostomy are prone to developing bacteremia, sepsis, recurrent pneumonia, and colonization with antibiotic resistant bacteria.[21] Recently, biofilms have been discovered on the inner surface of tracheostomy tubes. Bacteria in biofilms are resistant to standard antimicrobial agents.

The causative factors for wound infections often are the use of gauze and disinfectants as they induce secondary wound injury and prevent wound healing.[19] Use of fibrous wound dressings such as Aquacel (carboxy methylcellulose natrium sheet) and antimicrobial drain sponges (polyhexamethylene biguanide) can be used as adjuncts in controlling peristomal wound infections without disturbing the normal flora such as α-hemolytic streptococcus and *Staphylococcus epidermidis*).[19,21]

Paratracheal mediastinal abscess has also been described following tracheostomy.[22,23] This can be successfully treated with intravenous antibiotics and repeated aspirations of the abscess.[23] CT-guided percutaneous drainage of anterior mediastinal abscesses with a 16 F catheter has been described and could be a potential option for this complication, providing access without the morbidity associated with open surgery.[24] It is somewhat surprising that this complication does not occur more frequently, as the tracheostomy procedure may open the paratracheal space, through which the organisms may gain access to the mediastinum.

Subcutaneous Emphysema

The incidence of subcutaneous emphysema in patients undergoing tracheostomy ranges from 0 to 4%.[3] Air may be forced into the subcutaneous tissues during tracheostomy if the patient coughs a great deal when the trachea is open during the procedure or in the immediate postoperative period. This is more likely to occur in the following circumstances: if an uncuffed tracheostomy tube is used, the tracheostomy wound is closed with sutures, or the wound is packed when an uncuffed tube is used so that air escaping from the trachea is forced into the soft tissue planes around the wound.

Usually subcutaneous emphysema is mild and may be diagnosed by palpating crepitus in the tissues immediately surrounding the tracheostomy site. Occasionally extensive subcutaneous emphysema may cause the patient's entire body to be swollen because of air trapped in the soft tissues. Such massive subcutaneous emphysema and pneumomediastinitis has been reported to be caused by tracheostomy but resolved favorably over a 10-day period.[25]

Ironically, emergency tracheostomy is advocated in the management of subcutaneous emphysema developing from other causes. Recently, the placement of subcutaneous drains has been shown to be an effective, inexpensive, and safe way of providing effective decompression and resolution of subcutaneous emphysema. Other less effective techniques include insertion of medium- or large-bore intravenous catheters into the subcutaneous plane, or the use of multiple incisions or "blow holes" to help decompress the collected air.[26]

Subcutaneous emphysema can be prevented by three methods. The first is to secure the airway prior to the tracheostomy with an endotracheal tube or bronchoscope, which will prevent the high negative intrathoracic pressure that occurs while inspiring against an obstructed airway and promoting air dis-

section into the deep tissues and subsequently subcutaneous emphysema. The second method is to avoid excessive dissection of the pretracheal fascia and the tissues lateral to the trachea. The third method is to avoid closing the skin incision tightly around the tracheostomy tube. Closure of the wound or tightly packing around the wound can lead to dissection as high pressure air comes out of the tracheal incision and cannot escape through the skin incision. However, should this complication occur, the patient must be reassured that this situation is not serious and that it will usually resolve spontaneously within a few days as the trapped air is absorbed by the body. If the wound was sutured, the sutures should be removed, and any packing present should be removed. If an uncuffed tracheostomy tube was used, it should be replaced by a cuffed tube.

Swallowing Problems

Some patients may experience difficulties with swallowing after tracheostomy. Several explanations for this have been proposed: partial fixation of the vertical motion of the larynx, lack of laryngeal elevation, pressure of the cuff increasing pressure in the upper esophageal segment, reduction of laryngeal and hypopharyngeal sensitivity and alteration in the coughing mechanism, and loss of olfactory and gustatory stimulation of the swallowing process.[27] Conversely, dysphagia and laryngeal fixation lead the patient to swallow air, possibly to relieve a feeling of pressure in the throat; this in turn, may lead to gastric distention and discomfort.

Aspiration is another common swallowing disorder that accompanies tracheostomy. The mechanism for aspiration appears to be related to the mechanism for dysphagia. In addition, reduction in subglottic pressure, attenuation of the adductor vocal fold reflex, and a decrease in abductor vocal fold activity also contribute toward aspiration in patients who have a tracheostomy. The incidence of aspiration can range from 50 to 87%. There is a potential for the development of more serious complications such as aspiration pneumonia in these patients.[28]

Swallowing dysfunction usually resolves spontaneously, but the patient may be made more comfortable by insertion of a nasogastric tube to decompress the stomach, which may be distended by swallowed air. Swallowing function can be improved by deflating the cuff and placing a one-way speaking valve. Studies show that placing a one- way speaking valve such as a Passy-Muir valve facilitate swallowing (Fig 3–9) and reduce aspiration by improving laryngeal clearance, preventing laryngeal penetration and improving subglottic pressures.[29,30,31]

Aspiration also can be reduced by occlusion of the tracheostomy tube. Aspiration can be eliminated in 60% of patients and reduced in patients who continue to aspirate by tube occlusion. Unfortunately not all patients can withstand complete occlusion of the tube.[28] If a patient does aspirate, a cuffed tube should be inserted if not already in use and the patient should be suctioned often to remove secretions. An inflated cuff is not absolutely protective of the airway. Ding et al studied swallowing physiology in patients who have a tracheostomy with cuff inflated or deflated and found a greater incidence of silent aspiration and reduced laryngeal elevation in patients with cuff inflated.[32] This reiterates the importance of suctioning in patients with the tracheostomy tube

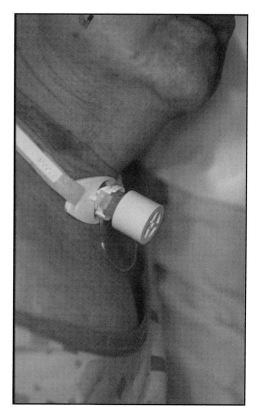

Fig 3-9. Patient with a tracheostomy tube with a Passy-Muir valve in place.

cuff inflated as the stagnant oral secretions have a potential to trickle down past the cuff into the trachea.

Tube Obstruction

Preventing obstruction of the tracheostomy tube begins with the procedure itself, which must be performed in such a way that the opening of the tube is not in contact with the anterior or posterior wall of the trachea. The surgeon also must be alert for the anatomic abnormalities that could lead to insertion of the tube into a blind pouch (as in cases of tracheoesophageal fistula repair) instead of into the tracheal lumen.

The tracheostomy tube may become obstructed by a blood clot or mucus. A mucus plug is a common cause of tube obstruction and may be fatal to the patient. This complication can be reduced by proper humidification of inspired air, the use of a tracheostomy tube with an inner cannula, and attentive nursing care. It is vitally important to remove the inner cannula frequently for cleaning, as mucus tends to collect at the tip of the tube and may dry and harden, thus occluding the lumen. Because an inner cannula usually is not used in children, it is especially important to ensure that the air is properly humidified and that suctioning and tube care are performed frequently enough to prevent the buildup of secretions.

Displaced Tracheostomy Tube

Causes. Displacement of the tracheostomy tube may occur at any time during or after the procedure. The tract between the skin and the trachea is usually not established until 5 or 6 days after the procedure and dislodgement of the tube before this time can be particularly dangerous. The tracheostomy tract matures over 10 to14 days and tube displacement thereafter is easier to manage.[33] Several factors may predispose to displacement of the tube, including: incorrect placement of the tube into the trachea during the tracheostomy, loosening of tapes as a result of resolution of subcutaneous emphysema or edema of the neck, excessive coughing, agitated movements of an uncooperative and confused patient, and an overweight or muscular patient with a large neck resulting in improper fit of the standard tracheostomy tube.[33,34]

Displacement of the tracheostomy tube may not always be apparent. If the tracheostomy was indicated for a complete upper airway obstruction, dislodgement of the tracheostomy tube will result in loss of the airway and respiratory obstruction, which can lead to respiratory arrest and death. However, if the patient has a partial upper airway obstruction, the displaced tube may not cause immediate and obvious respiratory distress.[34] Dislodgement should be suspected when a patient with a fresh tracheostomy has airway distress and a suction catheter cannot be passed through the tracheostomy tube into the trachea.

Prevention. The incidence of tracheostomy tube displacement is only about 1.5%; however, the mortality associated with it is very high. Factors that influence the outcome and management include the indication for the procedure, the patency of the upper airway, the time since the procedure was done, surgical technique, especially if traction sutures were used, and if there is a partial or complete dislodgement of the tube. In adults, the technique of tracheostomy affects the risk of decannulation and the ease of recannulation.[34] Removal of a portion of one tracheal ring between the second and fourth rings during the tracheostomy and making sure that the tube fits well and is positioned properly within the trachea reduces the risk of decannulation. In obese patients with a short, thick neck, the standard tracheostomy tube may not fit properly to the anatomy of these individuals. Accidental decannulation of an ill-fitting tracheostomy tube has been associated with increased morbidity and mortality. In such cases, special tracheostomy tubes may be used (see Fig 6–2, Chapter 6, Selecting a Tracheostomy Tube). Another viable option is "defatting" the skin flaps surrounding the stoma which helps reconturing the neck to accommodate a standard tube.[35] If the tube is secured with a tracheostomy tape or a Velcro strap, it should be tied around the neck (such that only one finger may be inserted between the tape and the skin of the neck) before the dressings are applied. Sutures should be used to anchor the neck plate of the tracheostomy tube to the skin for additional stability (see Fig 3–6). In addition, ventilator and oxygen-delivery tubing should be attached without tension and without exerting traction on the tracheostomy tube.

Management of the Displaced Tracheostomy Tube. When accidental decannulation occurs, it is most important that the tract be identified correctly to prevent the creation of a false passage when a new tube is inserted. This is aided by having adequate lighting and assistance to help with replacing the tube, by having the proper equipment (tracheostomy tray), by placing the patient in the position in which the procedure was performed (supine with extension of the neck), and by suctioning vigorously, but carefully, so that the tracheal lumen lines up with the stoma and can be identified with certainty. If traction sutures were placed in the tracheal rings just above and below the stoma at the time of the tracheostomy, traction on these sutures will both spread the skin edges and bring the stoma up to the level of the opening in the skin.[2] This makes it possible to maintain the airway until the tube is replaced and also makes reinsertion of the tube very accurate.

Under dire circumstances, when the tube displacement has been diagnosed and proper assistance, lighting, and instruments are not available, the tracheal fenestration can be identified digitally and the tube reinserted by feel. In some situations, an alternative to replacement of the tracheal tube is orotracheal intubation if the indication for the tracheostomy was not primarily related to upper airway obstruction.

After accidental decannulation, it is usually advisable to insert a tube a size smaller than the original tube so as not to traumatize the tissues. A suction catheter or flexible laryngoscope may be used as a guide for reinsertion of the tube: the new tube should be threaded over the catheter, the catheter placed into the lumen of the trachea, and the tube advanced carefully over the catheter. Fibreoptic tracheostomy guides, fibre optic bronchoscopes, or the Trachlight (originally developed to facilitate light-guided intubation techniques)[6] may be used in the same way and are particularly useful if the lumen of the trachea cannot be positively identified by direct inspection. After the new tube has been positioned, the patient should be ventilated and suctioned before the tracheostomy tapes or Velcro straps are secured.

Late Postoperative Complications

Granuloma Formation

The formation of a granuloma is more a consequence of tracheostomy than a complication of the procedure, as the wound is always moist and exposed to bacteria and some degree of mechanical irritation due to the motion of the tube. The incidence of granulation tissue formation is 10 to 80%.[36] Other possible causes of granulation tissue formation are bacterial infection, gastroesophageal reflux, and stents in tracheal graft procedures.[36] Initially granulation tissue is soft and vascular; but as the granuloma matures, it may become fibrous, and after a long period, become covered with epithelium. Such hard granulomas can form around the stoma, suprastomally within the trachea, and in the trachea at the tip of the tube. Granulation tissue can cause hemorrhage (especially in patients with altered coagulation profile), difficulty in replacing a dislodged tube, and delay in decannulation and may also result in obstruction of the tracheostomy tube or the trachea itself. In fact, obstruction related to granulation tissue has been cited as a cause of death in several patients.[36] These problems tend to be most common in children.

Granulation tissue and resultant granuloma may be seen when the tube is removed or can be appreciated on lateral radiographs. Although some granulomas resolve spontaneously, most must be treated. Meticulous skin care and the use of antimicrobial and corticosteroid preparations topically help to decrease bacterial contamination and the resultant inflammatory response leading to granulation tissue. Topical silver nitrate cauterization and inhaled beclamethasone has also been used for treating granulation tissue.[36]

Obstructing granulomas require surgical therapy. Several techniques may be used to remove these masses. If the granuloma is very soft, it may be removed endoscopically by scraping and suctioning out the mass with a velvet-eye suction through the stoma. Other approaches include using the endoscope and CO_2 or neodymium: yttrium aluminum garnet (Nd: YAG) laser to vaporize the granulation tissue.[37] When the granuloma is fibrous and covered with squamous epithelium, it may be necessary to excise the granulomas through an external, stomal, or a laryngofissure approach. Recently powered instrumentation tracheal surgery (PITS), namely, the microdebrider, has been shown to be beneficial in managing tracheal granulation tissue.[37]

Late Tracheoesophageal Fistula (TEF)

TEF occurs very rarely following tracheostomy, estimated as less than 1% of patients,[38] but may result when an overinflated or improperly fitted cuffed tube or a malpositioned tracheostomy cannula exerts pressure against an indwelling nasogastric tube. In addition, if the posterior wall of the trachea was penetrated during surgery and not repaired, a TEF could result. TEF may manifest as production of copious secretions, recurrent aspiration of food, increasing dyspnea, a persistent cuff leak, or severe gastric distention.[39] Diagnosis can be made with a contrast esophagography or CT scan of the mediastinum.[38,39]

If the mediastinum is involved in a secondary suppurative process, thoracotomy or CT-guided drainage may be necessary to drain the wound; however, if the process is localized in the neck, it may be drained through a cervical incision. Once the purulent exudate has been drained, the fistula may heal spontaneously with administration of antibiotics and attention to proper nutrition. If it does not heal spontaneously, placement of a stent in the esophagus and the trachea may alleviate the symptoms.

There are various options for surgical repair, the principle being identification and debridement of the fistulous tract and closure of the tract with interposition of soft tissue. Traditionally, TEF has been treated surgically through a lateral cervical incision with simple division and either direct closure or indirect (with interposition of soft tissue) closure of the fistula. The disadvantages of the lateral approach include a limited and unilateral exposure of the fistula, need for exposure of the left recurrent laryngeal nerve, and inadvertent esophageal rotation may lead to devascularization of the esophagus and consequently tracheal stenosis at the level of the repair.[38] The anterior approach described originally by Grillo et al,[40] which is a single-stage procedure involving tracheal resection and reanastomosis and a two-layer esophageal repair has been found to give excellent results in the surgical correction of TEF. This is a useful approach for the treatment of very large TEFs.[38,41]

Tracheocutaneous Fistula (TCF) and Depressed Scar

Failure of the tracheostomy stoma to close following decannulation is indicative of a tracheocutaneous fistula, the result of squamous epithelial surfaces of the skin and the trachea healing to one another. The incidence of TCF ranges from 3.3 to 42%.[42] This causes constant drainage from the fistula onto the neck as well as mucus being expelled when the patient coughs. The fistula occurs more often in the patient with a long-term tracheostomy and is always accompanied by a depressed scar. This scar is adherent to the trachea and attracts attention as the depressed scar moves when the patient swallows. Marked weight loss may predispose to TCF as the loss of subcutaneous tissue in the neck brings the skin closer to the trachea. The

incidence of TCF has reported to vary from less than 1% in patients who are decannulated quickly to more than 70% if the tracheostomy remains in place for over 16 weeks.[43] A higher incidence of TCF is noted in children who are treated with a "starplasty" technique of tracheostomy; and, hence, to a certain extent is dependent on the surgical technique.[44]

Persistent TCF can cause recurrent aspiration, infection, poor cough, skin irritation, and social and cosmetic nonacceptance.[42] The ideal treatment is closure of the fistula simply by excising the epithelium of the tract and allowing the tract to close by secondary intention. Closure occurs very rapidly and results in a watertight seal. This method is recommended for younger children in particular, because more extensive procedures may require lengthy anesthesia and the manipulation of the trachea could lead to edema and airway obstruction. This technique, although effective, leaves a depressed scar which may be revised at a later time.

Closure of the TCF may be facilitated by cautery or curettage; however, TCF that fail to close spontaneously within 6 months should be treated.[43] Myers described a technique in which the fistula is excised and the scar revised in a single-stage procedure.[45] The scar is excised through an elliptical incision placed at the level of and encompassing the depressed scar and the TCF (Fig 3–10A). The scar between the skin and the fistula is then released. The squamous epithelium of the fistula is left on the trachea and inverted into the stoma as a trap-door flap so that the trachea is lined with squamous epithelium. The skin superior and inferior to the incision is widely undermined. The strap muscles are usually incorporated in scar tissue and are adherent to the sides of the trachea (Fig 3–10B). The strap muscles are released and reapproximated in the midline (Fig 3–10C). Sewing the strap muscles together in the midline restores the normal anatomy, fills in the depressed scar and separates the trachea from the skin, thereby preventing the depressed scar, from reforming. The subcutaneous tissue should be closed without tension and without a drain and the skin closed with fast absorbing suture (Fig 3–10D).

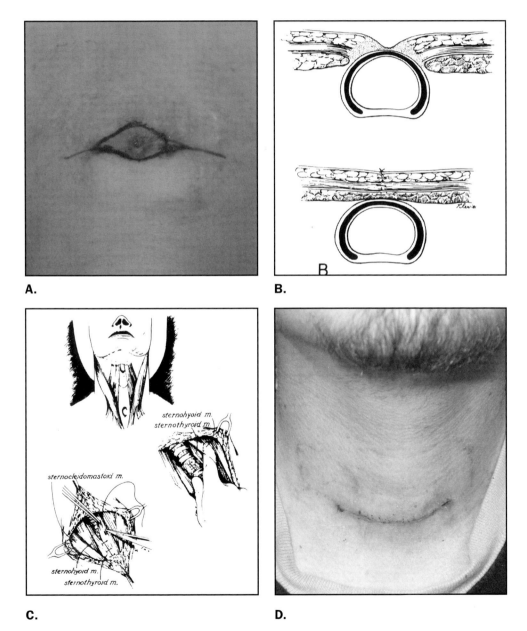

A.   **B.**

C.   **D.**

Fig 3-10. A. Depressed scar and tracheocutaneous fistula. **B.** Multilayer repair of a depressed scar. **C.** Multilayer repair. **D.** Normal appearance following scar revision

Steri-Strips and a fluff should be applied to the wound.

Potential complications of TCF closure include hematoma, infection, keloid formation, and subcutaneous emphysema.[43] Life-threatening subcutaneous emphysema has been reported following surgical repair of TCF which necessitated reopening of the tracheostomy.[42] Occasionally cervical emphysema may be the precursor of a focal air pocket that develops anterior to the trachea. This occurrence has been referred to as pneumatocele, pretracheal air cyst, tracheocele, and aerocele. Aeroceles are an unusual complication of TCF closure. Treatment includes simple drain placement, along with a pressure dressing, which can be performed as an outpatient procedure. In cases where the cyst presents months after TCF closure, the likelihood of mucosalization of the aerocele with formation of a true tracheocele is likely and requires a complete excision.[43]

Complications of TCF closure can be prevented by avoiding excessive coughing in the immediate postoperative period by extubating the patient when fully awake or by considering a short-term postoperative tracheal intubation to allow closure of the tracheal defect. In adults this procedure is usually done under local anesthesia with intravenous sedation to avoid the above. If crepitus is felt after the procedure, removal of a lateral skin suture along with a pressure dressing may prevent air entrapment.[42,43]

Laryngotracheal Stenosis

Tracheal stenosis following tracheostomy occurs in 0.6 to 21% of cases.[46] The trachea may become stenotic at the level of the stoma, the tip, or the cuff of the tracheostomy tube. Tracheal stenosis most often occurs at the area where the cuff of the tube rests as a result of ischemic injury from a high-pressure low-volume cuff which then leads to ischemia of the mucosa, ulceration, chondritis, cartilage necrosis, and scar. The use of high-volume low-pressure cuffs has markedly reduced the occurrence of such injuries.[46] Stenosis at the site of the stoma may be due to infection, chondritis of the peristomal tracheal cartilage, and the use of an excessively large tracheostomy tube or introduction of a large caliber tube into a small stoma by force.[46] Stomal stenosis is more likely to occur in patients whose tracheostomy tube is attached to a mechanical ventilator because the pistonlike motion of the tubing contributes to ulceration at the stoma. Stenosis at the tip of the tracheostomy tube, on the other hand, more often is due to the trauma caused as the tip of the tube rubs against the wall of the trachea, which may occur when the tube fits the trachea at an abnormal angle.

Although subglottic stenosis is often a complication of endotracheal intubation, it may occur following a high tracheostomy. The cricoid cartilage is vulnerable to injury. Children are more susceptible to subglottic stenosis because the cricoid cartilage is the narrowest part of the child's airway. The mechanism of subglottic stenosis is thought to be due to ischemia of the mucosa, chondritis from pressure injury to the cricoid cartilage, followed by bacterial infection, which leads to destruction of the cricoid cartilage and loss of cartilaginous support with scar formation, which narrows the airway.

Rigid bronchoscopy remains the procedure of choice for the evaluation of postintubation stenosis. However, there are many other options available for evaluation of the stenosis of the larynx and trachea, which include fiberoptic bronchoscopy, spiral CT scan which allows multiplanar reconstructions of the airway, and virtual bronchoscopy.[47] A recent study showed that virtual reality endobronchial simulation, VRES, using multidetector CT scanner was comparable to invasive bronchoscopy in the depiction of post-tracheostomy tracheal stenosis. VRES was more sensitive but less specific than invasive bronchoscopy. Although it could not detect granulations and synechiae due to lack of axial and multiplanar images, it was found to be helpful in selection of cases for more invasive treatments without the need for an invasive procedure.[48]

Prevention and Treatment. The best way to prevent tracheal stenosis is by using a high-volume low-pressure cuffed tracheostomy tube. The cuff should be deflated frequently to avoid ischemia of the tracheal mucosa. The patient should be fitted for an uncuffed tube as soon as appropriate. The tube must be of appropriate size and connected to any life-support systems in such a way that friction of the tube against the tracheal wall is minimized. Ideally a manometer should be used to prevent overinflation.

Tracheal stenosis is usually managed surgically, although conservative treatment methods such as repeated dilatations and endoscopic CO_2 laser ablation may be used if the stenosis is smaller that one tracheal ring or 1 cm in length with no circumferential scarring and no loss of cartilaginous support.[46,49] The stenotic segment usually involves more than one tracheal ring, and it is necessary to resect the stenotic portion of the trachea followed by an end-end anastomosis

(Fig 3–11A). The success rate of this procedure is reported to be 71 to 97%.[46]

The operation is carried out through a transcervical approach. After the strap muscles have been retracted, the stenotic area is identified (Fig 3–11B) and resected (Figs 3–11C and 3–11D) while taking care not to injure the recurrent laryngeal nerves. It is not necessary to resect the posterior membranous wall of the trachea, as it is usually not involved by stenosis. The superior and inferior tracheal rings are approximated with non-absorbable suture (Figs 3–11E, 3–11F, and 3–11G). The most common late complication after such surgery is the formation of granulation tissue at the suture line. These can be managed with endoscopic removal but Grillo has reported that they can be minimized with the use of absorbable suture material and with meticulous surgical technique.[50] Additional length of trachea to effect tension-free anastomosis may be obtained by mobilizing the laryngeal segment from the tongue base by transecting the suprahyoid muscles. Grillo described a method of gaining an even greater length of trachea by mobilizing the lung.[51] However, in a recent retrospective review of 901 patients of tracheal stenosis of whom 589 had postintubation stenosis, lengthy resection of the trachea were found to be fraught with failure. A safe limit of 4.5 cm of tracheal resection has been recommended to provide a tension-free anastomosis and to reduce the risk of anastomotic failure.[52]

Late Hemorrhage

Rupture of the innominate artery (creation of a tracheoinnominate fistula) is a rarely encountered but unfortunately an almost uniformly fatal complication

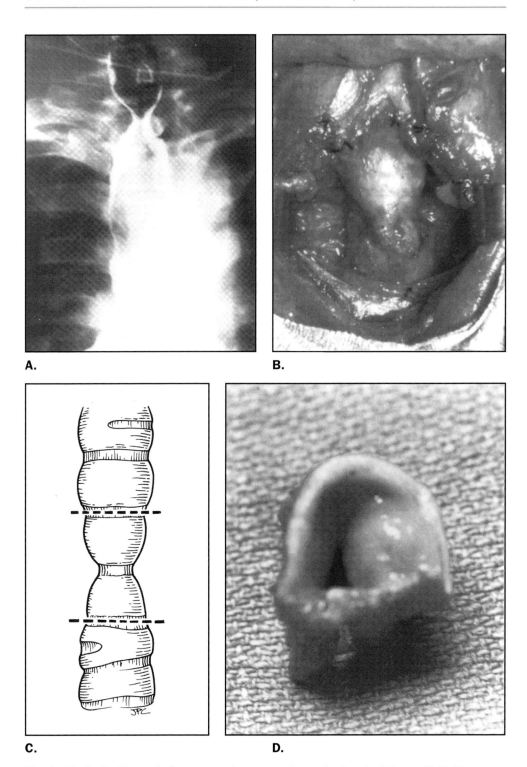

A.

B.

C.

D.

Fig 3–11. A. Radiograph demonstrating stenosis at the level of the cuff. **B.** The area of tracheal stenosis is identified. **C.** and **D.** The trachea is excised above and below the stenosis. **E.** An anode tube is inserted and the closure is begun. **F.** and **G.** Sutures are placed through the mucosa so that the knots are outside the lumen. *(Continues)*

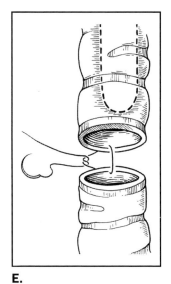 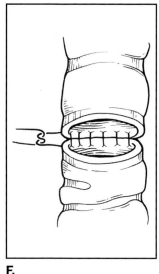 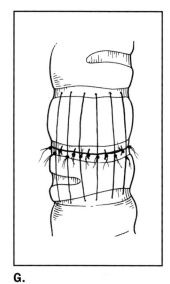

E. **F.** **G.**

Fig 3–11. *(Continued)*

occurring in 0.1 to 1% of all tracheostomies. It usually occurs between 3 days to 3 weeks postoperatively with a peak incidence between 7 to 14 days after the procedure. It is unusual for it to occur within the first 48 hours and bleeding occurring later than 3 weeks is usually secondary to granulation tissue, tracheobronchitis, or malignancy.[5]

There are several causative factors for this complication which can occur in any age group, such as:

1. Placing the tracheostomy too low on the trachea, below the third tracheal ring (Fig 3-12), where the pressure generated from the angulated neck of the tracheostomy tube can cause ischemic necrosis creating a communication between the anterior tracheal wall and the innominate artery;
2. An aberrant innominate artery which crosses the neck at the level of the cricoid cartilage can be damaged leading to catastrophic hemorrhage[53] (Fig 7-7);

3. Mechanical force from the tip of an excessively long or curved tube may erode the trachea and the vessel deep to it (see Fig.3-12);
4. Hyperextending the neck during the procedure may bring a high innominate artery artery into the field of dissection;
5. Prolonged pressure on the tracheal wall by an inflated cuff;
6. Infection of the trachea;
7. Administration of steroids.[5,45]

In 50% of cases, rupture of the innominate artery is usually heralded by a "sentinel bleed": the patient coughs up bright red (arterial) blood through the tracheostomy tube.[5] Initial management consists of maximum inflation of the cuff of the tracheostomy tube or digital pressure through the tracheostoma to tamponade the innominate artery.[5,54] In some cases, these maneuvers will successfully control the bleeding. If necessary the patient should be transfused while in transit to the operating room. Bronchoscopy is the diagnostic

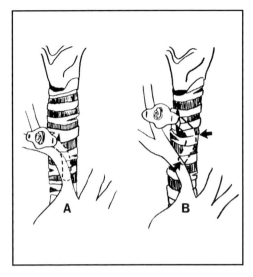
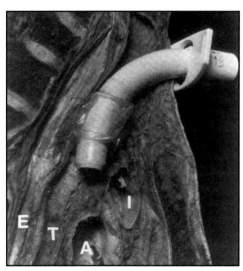

A.   **B.**   **C.**

Fig 3-12. A. The innominate artery was eroded by a tracheostomy tube placed too low in the trachea. **B.** Erosion of the innominate artery by a tube that was excessively long. **C.** Cadaver specimen showing a malpositioned tube with its tip pressing on the tracheal wall near innominate artery. (*I* = innominate artery; *A* = aorta; *T* = trachea; *E* = esophagus.)

procedure of choice; however, in the event of a massive hemorrhage, clinical suspicion warrants an emergency surgical exploration.[54] Standard surgical approach includes a median sternotomy with ligation of the innominate artery and drainage of the neck, with insertion of irrigation catheters to prevent mediastinitis. In specialized units, two separate incisions involving a right anterior thoracotomy and a neck approach may help prevent sternal split with prevention of mediastinitis and sternal dehiscence. Other successful surgical interventions have included the use of either saphenous or innominate vein grafts. Sternocleidomastoid patches or pedicled pericardial grafts also have been used. Whichever the approach or technique the goal of surgical intervention is terminating the flow in the innominate artery by debridement, transection, and ligation of the lumen. Ligation of the innominate artery has not been known to have any neurologic or vascular sequelae.[5] If the patient was being administered steroids, they must be discontinued.

SUMMARY

Most complications of tracheostomy can be prevented. Knowledge of the potential complications of tracheostomy is most important in preoperative planning and the use of specific techniques to prevent complications. Once recognized, the complication must be managed expeditiously to ensure the appropriate outcome.

REFERENCES

1. Henrich DE, Blythe WR, Weissler MC, Pillsbury HC. Tracheotomy and the intensive care unit patient. *Laryngoscope.* 1997;107:844-847.
2. Parnes SM, Myers EN. Traction sutures in a tracheostomy using a ligature passer. *Trans Am Acad Opthalmol Otolaryngol.* 1997;82:479.
3. Durbin CG Jr. Early complications of tracheostomy. *Resp Care.* 2005;50(4): 511-515.
4. Freeman BD, Isabella K, Lin N, Buchman TG. A meta-analysis of prospective trials comparing percutaneous and surgical tracheostomy in critically ill patients. *Chest.* 2000;118:1412-1418.
5. Grant CA, Dempsey G, Harrison J, Jones T. Tracheo-innominate artery fistula after percutaneous tracheostomy: three case reports and a clinical review. *Br J Anaesth.* 2006;96:127-131.
6. Mark DA. Identification of the obscured trachea using the Trachlight. *J Clin Anaesth.* 2005;17:235-237.
7. Marzelle J, Dartevelle P, Khalife J, Rojas-Miranda A, Chapelier A, Levasseur P. Surgical management of acquired post-intubation tracheo-oesophageal fistulas: 27 patients. *Eur J Cardiothorac Surg.* 1989; 3(6):499-502.
8. Kremer B, Botos-Kremer AI, Eckel HE, Schlondorff G. Indications, complications, and surgical techniques for pediatric tracheostomies—an update. *J Pediatr Surg.* 2002;37:1556-1562.
9. Jacobs JR, Thawley SE, Abata R, Sessions DG, Ogura JH. Posterior tracheal laceration: a rare complication of tracheostomy. *Laryngoscope.* 1978;88(12): 1942-1946.
10. Myers EN, Stool SE. Complications of tracheotomy. In: Myers EN, Stool SE, Johnson JT, eds. *Tracheotomy.* New York, NY: Churchill Livingstone, 1985:150.
11. Rabuzzi DD, Reed GF. Intrathoracic complications following tracheotomy in children. *Laryngoscope.* 1971;81:939.
12. Yamada M, Hirano M, Okhubo H. Recurrent laryngeal nerve paralysis: a 10-year review of 564 patients. *Auris Nasus Larynx.* 1983;10(suppl):S1-S15.
13. Kwon TK, Rosen CA, Gartner-Schmidt J. Preliminary results of a new temporary vocal fold injection material. *J Voice.* 2005;19(4):668-673.
14. Bosley B, Rosen CA, Simpson CB, McMullin BT, Gartner-Schmidt JL. Medial arytenoidectomy versus transverse cordotomy as a treatment for bilateral vocal fold paralysis. *Ann Otol Rhinol Laryngol.* 2005;114(12):922-926.
15. Jackson C, Jackson CL. *The Larynx and Its Diseases.* Philadelphia, Pa: WB Saunders; 1937.
16. Galvis AG, Stool SE, Bluestone CD. Pulmonary edema following relief of acute upper airway obstruction. *Ann Otol Rhinol Laryngol.* 1980:89:124-128.
17. Galvis AG. Pulmonary edema complicating relief of upper airway obstruction. *Am J Emerg Med.* 1987;5(4):294-297.
18. Oudjhane K, Bowen A, Oh KS, Young LW. Pulmonary edema complicating upper airway obstruction in infants and children. *Can Assoc Radiol J.* 1992;43(4): 278-282.
19. Tsunezuka Y, Suzuki M, Nitta K, Oda M. The use of fibrous wound dressing sheets made of carboxymethycellulose natrium in the postoperative management of tracheostomy. *Kyobu Geka.* 2005;58(12):1063-1067.
20. Snow N, Richardson JD, Flint LM. Management of necrotizing tracheostomy infections. *J Thorac Cardiovasc Surg.* 1981;82:341.
21. Motta GJ, Trigilia D. The effect of an antimicrobial drain sponge dressing on specific bacterial isolates at tracheostomy sites. *Ostomy Wound Manage.* 2005;51(1):60-62, 64-66.
22. Cole AG, Kerr JH. Paratracheal abscesses after tracheostomy. *Intens Care Med.* 1983;9:345.
23. Watanakunakorn C. Successful novel drainage treatment of mediastinal abscess

complicating tracheostomy. *Chest*. 1989; 96(4):946-948.

24. Gevenois PA, Sergent G, De Myttenaere M, Beernaerts A, Rocmans P. CT-guided percutaneous drainage of an anterior mediastinal abscess with a 16 F catheter. *Eur Respir J*. 1995;8(5):869-870.

25. Rivares Esteban JJ, Gil Paraiso PJ, Navarro Diaz F, Martin Martin JM, Campos del Alamo MA, Marin Garcia J. Subcutaneous cervico-thoracic emphysema and pneumomediastinum following a tracheostomy. *An Otorrinolaringol Ibero Am*. 2001; 28(6):599-605.

26. Sherif HM, Ott DA. The use of subcutaneous drains to manage subcutaneous emphysema. *Tex Heart Inst J*. 1999; 26(2):129-131.

27. Martin F. Dysphagia due to tracheotomy. *Med Klin*. 1999;94:43-44.

28. Suiter DM, McCullough GH, Powell PW. Effects of cuff deflation and one-way tracheostomy speaking valve placement on swallow physiology. *Dysphagia*. 2003; 18(4):284-292.

29. Dettelbach MA, Gross RD, Mahimann J, Eibling DE. Effect of the Passy-Muir valve on aspiration in patients with tracheostomy. *Head Neck*. 1995;17(4): 297-302.

30. Ohmae Y, Adachi Z, Isoda Y, et al. Effects of one-way speaking valve placement on swallowing physiology for tracheostomized patients impact on laryngeal clearance. *Nippon Jibiinkoka Gakkai Kaiho*. 2006;109(7):594-599.

31. Gross RD, Mahimann J, Grayhack JP. Physiologic effects of open and closed tracheostomy tubes on the pharyngeal swallow. *Ann Otol Rhinol Laryngol*. 2003;112(2):143-152.

32. Ding R, Longemann JA. Swallow physiology in patients with trach cuff inflated or deflated: a retrospective study. *Head Neck*. 2005;27(9):809-813.

33 Rajendram R, McGuire N. Repositioning a displaced tracheostomy tube with an Aintree intubation catheter mounted on a fibre-optic bronchoscope. *Br J Anaesth*. 2006;97(4):576-579.

34. Seay SJ, Gay SL. Problem in tracheostomy patient care: recognizing the patient with a displaced tracheostomy tube. *ORL Head Neck Nurs*.1997;15(2):10-11.

35. Gross ND, Cohen JI, Andersen PE, Wax MK. "Defatting" tracheostomy in morbidly obese patients. *Laryngoscope*. 2002;112:1940-1944.

36. Yaremchuk K. Regular tracheostomy tube changes to prevent formation of granulation tissue. *Laryngoscope*. 2003;113:1-10.

37. Fang TJ, Lee LIA, Li HY. Powered instrumentation in the treatment of tracheal granulation tissue for decannulation. *Oto-laryngol Head Neck Surg*. 2005; 133(4):520-524.

38. Epstein SK. Late complications of tracheostomy. *Respir Care*. 2005;50(4): 542-549.

39. Sue RD, Susanto I. Long-term complications of artificial airways. *Clin Chest Med*. 2003;24(3):457-471.

40. Grillo HC, Moncure AC, McEnany MT. Repair of inflammatory tracheoesophageal fistula. *Ann Thorac Surg*. 1976; 22:112-119.

41. Oliara A, Rena O, Papalia E, Filosso PL, Ruffini E, Pischedda F, Cavallo A, Maggi G. Surgical management of acquired nonmalignant tracheo-esophageal fistulas. *J Cardiovasc Surg*. 2001;42(2):257-260.

42. Mohan VK, Kashyap L, Verma S. Life threatening subcutaneous emphysema following surgical repair of tracheocutaneous fistula. *Paediatr Anaesth*. 2003; 13(4):339-341.

43. Bent JP 3rd, Smith RJ. Aerocele after tracheocutaneous fistula closure. *Int J Pediatr Otorhinolaryngol*. 1998;42(3):257-261.

44. Sautter NB, Krakovitz PR, Solares CA, Koltai PJ. Closure of persistent tracheocutaneous fistula following "starplasty" tracheostomy in children. *Int J Pediatr Otorhinolaryngol*. 2006;70(1):99-105.

45. Myers EN, Stool SE. Complications of tracheotomy. In: Myers EN, Stool SE, John-

son JT, eds. *Tracheotomy*. New York, NY: Churchill Livingstone; 1985:161–164.

46. Sarper A, Ayten A, Eser I, Ozbudak O, Demircan A. Tracheal stenosis after tracheostomy or intubation: review with special regard to cause and management. *Tex Heart Inst J.* 2005;32(2): 154–158.

47. Carretta A, Melloni G, Ciriaco P, et al. Preoperative assessment in patients with postintubation tracheal stenosis: rigid and flexible bronchoscopy versus spiral CT scan with multiplanar reconstructions. *Surg Endosc.* 2006;20(6):905–908.

48. Joshi AR, Khanna PC, Merchant SA, Khandelwal A, Agrawal N, Karnik ND. Role of multidetector CT virtual bronchoscopy in the evaluation of post-tracheostomy tracheal stenosis—a preliminary study. *J Assoc Physicians India.* 2003;51:871–876.

49. Myers EN. Tracheal resection and anastomosis. In: Myers EN, ed. *Operative Otolaryngology-Head and Neck Surgery.* Philadelphia, Pa: WB Saunders; 1997: 592–596.

50. Grillo HC. Management of nonneoplastic diseases of the trachea. In: Shields TW, LoCicero J III, Ponn RB, eds. *General Thoracic Surgery.* Vol 1. 5th ed. Philadelphia, Pa: Lippincott Williams & Wilkins; 2000:885–897.

51. Grillo HC. The management of tracheal stenosis following assisted respiration. *J Thorac Cardiovasc Surg.* 1969;57:52.

52. Wright CD, Grillo HC, Wain JC, et al. Anastomotic complications after tracheal resection: prognostic factors and management. *J Thorac Cardiovasc Surg.* 2004;128(5):731–739.

53. Ozlugedik S, Ozcan M, Unal A, Yalcin F, Tezer MS. Surgical importance of highly located innominate artery in neck surgery. *Am J Otolaryngol.* 2005;26(5): 330–332.

54. Allan JS, Wright CD. Tracheoinnominate fistula: diagnosis and management. *Chest Surg Clin N Am.* 2003;13(2):331–341.

CHAPTER 4

Technique and Complications of Tracheostomy in the Pediatric Age Group

ROBERT F. YELLON

PREOPERATIVE PLANNING

A decision to perform a tracheostomy in an infant or child should be made carefully, as this decision has a major, far-reaching impact with significant medical, family, and financial implications. The mean hospital stay following tracheostomy in an infant or child is 50 days with an average cost of $200,000.[1] Parents caring for a child with a tracheotomy experience significant caregiver burden including reduced mental health status which worsens relative to the child's severity of illness and the increasing costs.[2] In one study of 181 children who underwent a tracheostomy,[3] 64% were eventually decannulated, but the average length of tracheostomy use was 365 days during the 5-year study period. The major indications for tracheostomy were airway obstruction (60%), prolonged ventilatory support (30%), and the need for pulmonary toilet (10%).

Communication between the surgeon and the anesthesiologist is critical prior to performing a tracheostomy in a child. Primary and contingency plans for securing the airway must be developed and agreed upon. The patient should be examined for anatomic problems that might possibly lead to difficult endotracheal intubation, such as mandibular hypoplasia, macroglossia, prolapse of the base of the tongue, or the presence of a pharyngeal or laryngotracheal mass. The patient's history of previous intubation, laryngoscopy, or bronchoscopy should be obtained to anticipate difficulties. Flexible nasopharyngolaryngoscopy, direct laryngoscopy, rigid bronchoscopy, and possibly esophagoscopy are important examinations to help determine the exact reasons for airway obstruction, intractable aspiration, or the need for prolonged ventilatory support. Information derived from these examinations will be an aid in the decision-making process for or against tracheostomy in a child.

If possible, tracheostomy should be performed in the operating room where there are enough personnel to assist as well as adequate lighting, suction, surgical equipment, tracheostomy tubes, endotracheal tubes, and rigid bronchoscopes. A wide range of tracheostomy tubes, endotracheal tubes, and laryngoscopes of appropriate sizes must be available.

Establishment of an artificial airway in a child with a tenuous airway should be strongly considered before the child depletes all of his or her respiratory reserve and progresses to complete obstruction or respiratory failure, which will result in a high-risk emergency tracheostomy.[4] Planned elective tracheostomy with a secured airway, is preferred over a hurried emergency tracheostomy performed during acute severe airway obstruction with oxyhemoglobin desaturations. In extreme circumstances, cricothyroidotomy may be required.

Securing the airway by initial direct laryngoscopy or flexible tracheobronchoscopy followed by endotracheal intubation, or with a rigid bronchoscope that is subsequently converted to tracheostomy is strongly recommended to avoid possible sudden airway obstruction.[4] The patient is anesthetized for the tracheostomy after the airway has been secured.

Unsuccessful attempts at intubation may also precipitate acute airway obstruction; thus tracheostomy under local anesthesia has occasionally been performed. Selected patients, such as older, cooperative children with penetrating laryngeal trauma in which positive-pressure ventilation would risk subcutaneous emphysema or pneumothorax, may be appropriate subjects for tracheostomy under local anesthesia.

Position of Patient

The patient should be placed on the operating table with a rolled towel or blanket under the shoulders to extend the neck. The anesthesiologist lifts the chin superiorly to provide maximal exposure. Extension of the neck in a patient with a cervical fracture may be fatal and is contraindicated. In a patient with scoliosis it may not be possible to extend the neck. The procedure is more difficult and poses a higher risk in such patients.

TECHNIQUE OF TRACHEOSTOMY

The landmarks of the midline, hyoid bone, thyroid notch, cricoid cartilage, thyroid isthmus, and sternal notch are identified by palpation and the skin incision marked appropriately. It should be noted that the hyoid bone, thyroid cartilage, and cricoid are positioned superiorly in the infant's neck as compared with that of the adult. Nasogastric tubes or esophageal stethoscopes must be removed, as their presence in the esophagus may lead to mistaking the esophagus for the trachea, thereby increasing the risk of iatrogenic esophageal injury.

Lidocaine 0.05% with epinephrine solution 1:100,000 is infiltrated into the planned 1.5-cm horizontal incision line. If possible, the incision is made a minimum of one finger's breadth above the sternal notch but below the thyroid isthmus. If the incision is made too close to the sternal notch, the trachea is difficult to identify. Another problem is that an incision placed too low on the neck may leave a stretched and unsightly scar. The skin is incised and the underlying fat removed to give good exposure of the middle layer of the deep cervical fascia overlying the strap muscles. After the midline raphe is identified, the surgeon and assistant each grasp the medial edge of the strap muscles and lift, separate, and divide the muscles along the raphe. As the dissection proceeds to a deeper layer, it is advisable to place the right-angle blunt end of Senn retractors on either side of the trachea to improve exposure and to protect the anterior jugular veins. The successive layers of strap muscles and connective tissue are divided in this manner. Deep dissection without good exposure should be avoided as difficult to control bleeding may occur.

The pretracheal fascia is identified and gently incised. Care must be taken to avoid excessive dissection lateral to the trachea to decrease the possibility of dissection of air into the tissues and pneumothorax. If the thyroid isthmus cannot be retracted superiorly, it may be divided with electrocautery for infants or suture-ligated in older children to avoid bleeding.

The same lidocaine with epinephrine solution may be infiltrated into the planned vertical incision in the trachea to decrease mucosal bleeding. This incision is generally made through two or three tracheal rings, usually within the second to fifth tracheal rings. An incision close to the cricoid should be avoided, as this is associated with a greater chance of development of subglottic stenosis.

Nylon traction sutures are placed in the trachea on either side of the incision line before the incision is made, and a second pair of traction sutures is placed along the cut edge of the trachea after the incision is made. These sutures are useful for retraction and are very helpful in locating the tracheostomy incision if accidental decannulation occurs in the early postoperative period.[5] The vertical incision in the trachea should be long enough to admit the tracheostomy tube easily. A small incision or a horizontal incision may lead to suprastomal collapse of the tracheal ring above the tube into the airway as the curved tube exerts pressure on this tracheal ring.

The endotracheal tube or bronchoscope is slowly withdrawn to a position just above the level of the incision but left in the airway until the tracheostomy tube is inserted and secured. Twill tracheostomy tapes are then placed and tied with the infant's head in a flexed position. The traction sutures are tied loosely with a loop and taped to the skin of the anterior chest. Tape labels are used that state clearly, "*traction sutures—do not remove.*" The incision is usually not sutured or packed to avoid subcutaneous emphysema. If the tracheostomy is expected to be permanent the tracheal cartilage may be sutured directly to the skin of the stoma or a trap-door tracheal flap may be sutured to the skin to create a permanent tracheostomy.

An alternative to standard tracheostomy is "starplasty"[6] of the stoma with alternating triangular skin and cartilage flaps which are sewn together to create a funnel-shaped mucocutaneous suture line. This technique has the advantage of decreased incidence of pneumothorax and easy reinsertion of the tube following accidental decannulation. The disadvantage of this technique is the high incidence of persistent tracheocutaneous fistula following planned decannulation.[7]

The position of the tracheostomy tube with respect to the carina and tracheal wall may be determined either by passing a small-diameter pediatric flexible endoscope through the tube (Fig 4–1) or by a chest radiograph (Fig 4–2). The postoperative radiograph will also identify pneumothorax or pneumomediastinum, if present. There are proponents for[8] and against[9] the use of routine post-tracheostomy chest radiographs. The author feels strongly that, although some series of pediatric post-tracheostomy

patients have reported many negative chest radiographs, the cost, morbidity, and possible mortality of missing one sig-

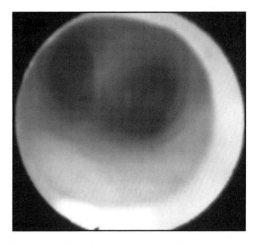

Fig 4–1. Flexible fiberoptic view through the tracheostomy tube that shows good tube position approximately 1 cm from carina.

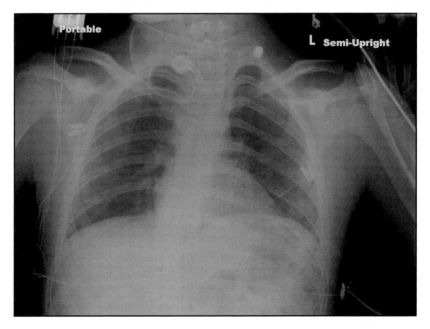

Fig 4–2. Chest radiograph of a child following a tracheostomy who experienced repeated accidental early decannulation. The radiograph shows a tracheostomy tube that is too short and barely reaches the trachea.

nificant post-tracheostomy complication that would have been identified on the chest radiograph will negate any savings from not performing the study.

In general, the tip of the tracheostomy tube should be 5 to 20 mm from the carina. When necessary, a standard-size tracheostomy tube may be carefully cut to a shorter length and the sharp edges beveled. This can be used until a specially ordered custom length tube arrives. The tube should also not be so short that the lumen faces the posterior wall of the trachea or is at risk to fall out easily (Figs 4–2 and 4–3). Certain patients, such as those with metabolic storage diseases or obese patients, may have excessive tissue between the skin and the trachea; thus a special long tracheostomy tube such as a custom Shiley (Mallinkrodt Medical, St. Louis, Mo) tube or a long or adjustable Bivona (Bivona Medical Technology, Gary, Ind) (Fig 4–4) tube may be required to achieve adequate tube length and to avoid accidental decannulation.

The long adjustable Bivona tube is later replaced by a custom ordered nonadjustable tube with the proper length. Special Bivona "Hyperflex"™ tracheostomy tubes (Fig 4–5) that are very useful for the

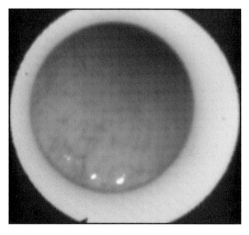

Fig 4–3. Flexible fiberoptic view through the tracheostomy tube that shows that the tube is too short and impinges on the posterior tracheal wall with partial obstruction of the tube.

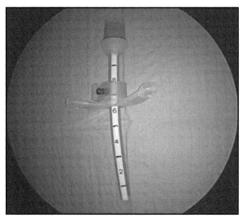

A.

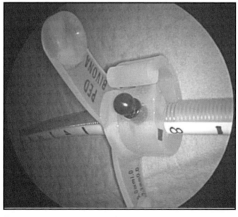

B.

Fig 4–4. Bivona Adjustable Flange Hyperflex™ Pediatric Tracheostomy Tube. **A.** This tube has an adjustable neck flange that allows the length of the tube to be changed based on the special needs of the individual patient. **B.** This tube is particularly useful for patients with a very thick neck who require an extra long tracheostomy tube.

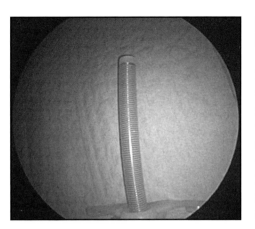

Fig 4–5. The Bivona Hyperflex™ Pediatric Tracheostomy Tube is very useful for patients with a tortuous tracheas such as those with severe scoliosis. As the tube is noncompressible but highly flexible, it gently conforms to the trachea but is atraumatic and will not erode the trachea.

patient with a tortuous trachea, such as patients with severe scoliosis, may also be ordered. This special ordered tube with a wire coil inside is noncompressible, but highly flexible. Thus, this tube conforms nicely to the tortuous trachea without causing trauma that would have been caused by more rigid tubes. Bivona tracheostomy tubes may also be ordered with an extended flange (Flextend™) that brings the connector away from the neck. This type of tube is very useful for patients with redundant anterior neck tissue.

If an innominate vessel is encountered overlying the trachea at the planned tracheostomy site, an incision may be made at a different level to avoid the vessel. If it is not possible to choose a second location, the vessel may be protected from erosion by the tracheostomy tube by covering the vessel with a local flap of strap or sternocleidomastoid muscle, which is sutured to the trachea and surrounding muscles.

EMERGENCY TRACHEOSTOMY

In extreme circumstances, a cricothyroidotomy may be performed as a lifesaving measure. A tracheostomy tube or an endotracheal tube may be placed temporarily and a formal tracheostomy carried out when the patient's condition has stabilized. Formal tracheostomy should be performed as soon as possible (<24 hours) as prolonged cricothyroidotomy and high tracheostomy are associated with development of subglottic stenosis.

A large-bore catheter (eg, 14-gauge) may also be useful when placed through the cricothyroid membrane into the airway to allow insufflation of oxygen until an endotracheal tube or tracheostomy tube is placed.

POSTOPERATIVE CARE

The patient should be closely observed for at least 5 days in the intensive care unit. Humidified air should be delivered via a tracheostomy collar, and frequent suctioning must be performed. Personnel caring for the child should be instructed in the use of the traction sutures following accidental early decannulation as well as standard procedures for changing the tracheostomy tube. Feedings may be resumed after 1 to 2 days.

Usually after 5 days, the stoma is mature and the first planned tube change is performed by the surgical staff. Allowing time for the stoma to heal and mature decreases the chances of a false passage of the tracheostomy tube to a position outside the trachea. Changing the tracheostomy tube is optimally performed by two trained individuals, with the child's neck extended, good lighting, and sterile conditions. The original tube is removed and a new tube is inserted.

Alternatively, the tube may be changed over a suction catheter with the hub cut off, which is then placed through the tracheostomy tube into the trachea while the outer end of the suction catheter is held securely. The tracheostomy tube is removed while the catheter is left in the stoma and trachea and the new tube is threaded over the catheter into the trachea. Thus, the suction catheter is used as a guide over which the new tracheostomy tube is changed. The traction sutures are removed after the first tracheostomy tube change. The patient is then transferred to a regular room with appropriate monitoring devices such as apnea and bradycardia monitors or pulse oximetry. Finally, the parents and other caretakers are instructed in tracheostomy care and cardiopulmonary resuscitation.

Once the caretakers have been trained, all necessary tracheostomy care equipment is in place in the home, and the patient's condition is otherwise satisfactory, the patient may be discharged.[10] The tracheostomy tube is generally changed once a week unless plugging of the tube requires that it be changed more often. The local emergency services personnel should be notified as to the child's presence in the community, as should the telephone and power companies, in order to give the child's home priority for repairs and emergencies.

COMPLICATIONS OF TRACHEOSTOMY

Complications are best prevented by careful preoperative planning, excellent communication between the surgeons and anesthesiologist, meticulous attention to detail intraoperatively, and careful long-term care. Even under optimum conditions complications may still occur.

INTRAOPERATIVE COMPLICATIONS

Hemorrhage

A careful history of abnormal bleeding or easy bruising in the patient or family must be sought. A history of ingestion of anticoagulants, aspirin, or other nonsteroidal anti-inflammatory drugs should be determined. In selected patients, screening or formal coagulation studies may be ordered and abnormalities corrected, when possible, prior to the tracheostomy.

Vascular structures such as the anterior jugular veins, thyroid isthmus, and innominate arteries and veins must be identified and ligated, moved, or covered with muscle flaps if necessary. Bleeding may occur following a paroxysm of coughing or after restoration of normal blood pressure following hypotension. The airway should again be secured via endotracheal tube or rigid bronchoscopy and the tracheostomy tube removed to allow retraction, suctioning, and visualization of the vessel in the stoma for definitive control of hemorrhage.

Air Dissection

Dissection of air in the deep paratracheal tissues is the cause of subcutaneous emphysema, pneumothorax, or pneumomediastinum. There are three methods to decrease dissection of air into the soft tissues. The first is to secure the airway prior to the tracheostomy with an endotracheal tube or bronchoscope, which will prevent the high negative intrathoracic pressure that occurs as the child inspires against an obstructed airway and promotes air dissection into the deep tissues. The second method is to avoid excessive dissection of the pretracheal fascia and the tissues lateral to the trachea. The third method is to avoid closing the skin incision tightly around the tracheostomy tube. Closure of the wound can lead to air dissection as high-pressure air comes out of the tracheal incision and cannot escape through the skin incision.

The treatment of air dissection is usually expectant, with careful observation. The tracheostomy skin incision should be left open or widened if it is too narrow. Occasionally, insertion of a chest tube may be necessary.

Iatrogenic Trauma

Care must be taken to avoid injury to several vital structures. The cricoid cartilage must not be injured as injury to the cricoid may lead to chondronecrosis and subglottic stenosis. If possible, the tracheal incision should be placed at least two rings below the cricoid cartilage. Avoidance of dissection lateral to the trachea should prevent damage to the recurrent laryngeal nerves. In an infant, the dome of the pleura may extend into the inferior aspect of the neck and inadvertent laceration may cause pneumothorax.

At the time of the tracheal incision, special care must be taken to avoid lacerating the posterior wall of the trachea and esophagus. Having a bronchoscope or endotracheal tube in the trachea will help to protect the posterior wall of the trachea and esophagus. Nasogastric tubes or esophageal stethoscopes should be removed. An iatrogenic tracheoesoph-

ageal fistula should be repaired as soon as the airway is secured. It is advisable, in this situation, to place a muscle flap between the trachea and esophagus to reinforce the closure.

Tracheostomy Tube Problems

A tube that is too short may fall out or become obstructed against the posterior wall of the trachea (see Figs 4-2 and 4-3); a tube that is too long may cause excessive coughing as it touches the carina, or the right mainstem bronchus may be intubated. Children with significant scoliosis or other deformities may have deviation of the trachea, which requires use of a custom made very flexible tracheostomy tube such as the Bivona Hyperflex tube (Bivona Medical Technologies, Gary, Ind), which easily conforms to the contour of the trachea (see Fig 4-5).

Cardiopulmonary Arrest

Relief of hypercarbia after tracheostomy may result in arrhythmias, hypotension, and apnea. Relief of hypoxia following a tracheostomy may also cause loss of drive of the respiratory center.[11] Other causes include a tracheostomy tube that is too short or too long or that has been placed into a false passage in the paratracheal position.

Postobstructive Pulmonary Edema

Postobstructive pulmonary edema may occur in a child who has had chronic or subacute upper airway obstruction. The high negative intrathoracic inspiratory pressure serves to increase pulmonary interstitial water, as does hypercarbia with pulmonary hypertension. During an episode of laryngospasm, the excessively high negative intrathoracic inspiratory pressure causes the interstitial fluid to enter the alveoli.[12] Positive-pressure ventilation is the appropriate treatment, although some also advocate the use of diuretics.

EARLY POSTOPERATIVE COMPLICATIONS

Hemorrhage

Bleeding may occur when the vasoconstriction from the lidocaine/epinephrine solution wears off. Prolonged oozing may be due to a coagulopathy and must be investigated. Mild bleeding may be controlled by *loose* packing of the incision. More significant bleeding should be addressed by returning the patient to the operating room, securing the airway, exploring the wound, and identifying and controlling the bleeding vessels.

Wound Infection

Although the tracheostomy always becomes colonized within 24 hours, occasionally cellulitis may occur, as may pneumonia or tracheitis. Meticulous hand washing and sterile technique help to decrease these problems, but they may still arise. Culture-directed antimicrobial treatment is indicated for a true infection, but not for a colonized stoma. The offending organisms are frequently resistant to first-line antimicrobial agents and

thus early culture and sensitivity specimens of purulent tracheostomy secretions should be obtained.[13] Recently, bacterial biofilms have been detected on the inner surfaces of tracheostomy tubes. Bacteria in biofilms are resistant to standard antimicrobial agents and may possibly be a potential source of pulmonary infection in patients with a tracheostomy tube.[14]

Swallowing Problems

Dysphagia may follow tracheostomy due to partial fixation of the vertical motion of the larynx by the tube. Excessive swallowing of air may lead to gastric dilation, which will require decompression with a nasogastric tube. Aspiration may occur, possibly due to the loss of the laryngeal closure reflex that follows tracheostomy.[15] A cuffed tracheostomy tube and frequent suctioning may minimize, but not completely prevent, tracheobronchial aspiration. Flexible fiberoptic laryngoscopy is indicated to assess for vocal cord immobility. Unilateral vocal cord paralysis may be treated by injection of the various substances lateral to the vocal cord or open thyroplasty. Aspiration in a child with a tracheostomy also may be successfully prevented with the use of continuous positive airway pressure (CPAP) applied to the tube.[16] Tracheal CPAP creates a pressure gradient that prevents aspiration into the lower airway. Intractable aspiration may require laryngotracheal separation.

Obstruction of the Tracheostomy Tube

A tube that is too short (see Fig 4–3) or too long may become obstructed by the posterior or anterior wall of the trachea, respectively. In the case of repaired tracheoesophageal fistula, care must be taken to avoid placing the tip of the tracheostomy tube into the blind pouch of the fistula repair.

Plugging of the tracheostomy tube may occur from blood clot; thick, tenacious mucus; or dried secretions. This complication may be minimized by humidification of inspired air and frequent suctioning and saline irrigation of the trachea and tube. The inner cannula should be changed and cleaned frequently. A tube without an inner cannula should be changed at least once a week or more frequently if necessary.

Accidental Decannulation

Life-threatening displacement of the tube may occur at any time but is most dangerous in the first 5 days following tracheostomy before a mature tract has formed around the tube. This is why patients should be observed in the intensive care unit for at least 5 days following tracheostomy and until the first tube change.

This complication may be prevented by selecting a tube that is not too short, especially in patients who have excessive soft tissue between the skin and the trachea. Tying the tracheostomy tube ties securely to admit only one finger under the ties is important. Suturing the neck plate of the tracheostomy tube to the skin also may be helpful in preventing accidential decannulation. Ventilator and oxygen tubing must be secured to the tube without tension. Uncooperative patients may require sedation or restraints to prevent them from pulling out the tube.

The use of traction sutures on either side of the tracheostomy incision has been an important method for identifying the tracheostomy incision to allow successful reinsertion of the tube following accidental decannulation.[5] Adequate suctioning and lighting are important. If passage of the usual size tube is difficult, a smaller tube, which should always be available, should be passed. Passing the tube over a suction catheter or a flexible bronchoscope are other important alternatives. This minimizes the chances of a false passage of the tube into a paratracheal site.

LATE COMPLICATIONS

Granuloma Formation

A suprastomal granuloma frequently forms at the superior aspect of the internal tracheal stoma. These granulomas may bleed, and also may prevent successful decannulation. Small, soft granulomas may be removed endoscopically, in the operating room or under direct vision through the stoma with hooks and hemostats, a sphenoid punch, or an endoscopically guided forceps.[17,18] Another option for removal of these lesions is the use of the KTP (potassium titanyl phosphate) or YAG laser fiber passed through a rigid bronchoscope.[19]

For a large, obstructing or fibrous suprastomal granuloma, it may be necessary to open the trachea directly.[17,18] Complete aphonia in a child with a tracheostomy who previously had a voice may indicate the presence of a totally obstructing suprastomal granuloma. Gastroesophageal reflux and bacterial infection are often present in these cases and should be treated appropriately,[17] which may possibly help to reduce the size and recurrence of these lesions. One study suggested that removal of the granulomas was associated with a greater chance of their return.[20] Thus, it may be wise to only remove large obstructing granulomas,[17,18] and those that are present just prior to decannulation.

Suprastomal Collapse

Collapse of the tracheal rings above the tracheostomy tube into the lumen of the trachea is usually minor but may occasionally be severe enough to cause significant airway obstruction and prevent decannulation. In severe cases, the obstructing tissue may require elevation or excision. The suprastomal collapse may be excised endoscopically using a KTP or ND:YAG laser fiber after a metal tracheostomy tube has been placed.[21] Open elevation or excision of the obstructing tissue also may be useful, as is reconstruction with cartilage grafting.

Tracheoesophageal Fistula

Late tracheoesophageal fistulas may follow tracheostomy. This problem is more likely to occur when a large-bore nasogastric tube is used especially in conjunction with a cuffed tracheostomy tube, as ischemic injury and necrosis of the soft tissue occurs between the tubes. An excessively large or long tube also may cause this problem. A small fistula may be treated by removal of the offending tubes and drainage of the wound. A large fistula may require interposition of a soft tissue flap between the trachea and the esophagus.

Tracheal and Subglottic Stenosis

Stenosis may occur at the level of the subglottis, the suprastomal area, the area at the tracheostomy tube cuff, or the tip of the tube. The factors that are believed to contribute to laryngotracheal stenosis include trauma,[22] bacterial infection,[23] and gastroesophageal reflux.[24] High tracheostomy incision with injury to the cricoid cartilage, when associated with bacterial infection and chondritis, can lead to subglottic stenosis. The cartilage ring above the stoma may prolapse into the lumen, thereby causing obstruction. Use of a low-volume, high-pressure cuff with excessively high pressures can cause ischemic necrosis of the mucosa, ulceration, chondritis, and ultimately stenosis. The tip of a poorly fitting tube may cause local trauma and possibly lead to tracheal stenosis.

Early stenosis may respond to treatment with antimicrobial agents, corticosteroids, and appropriate treatment of gastroesophageal reflux. Small, mature lesions may respond to dilation or laser excision. More extensive lesions will require excision and end-to-end anastomosis or formal laryngotracheal reconstruction with grafting.

Erosion of the Innominate Artery (Tracheoinnominate Artery Fistula)

Erosion of the tracheostomy tube into the innominate artery is often fatal. The artery may be eroded by a tracheostomy tube when the tube contacts the artery by (1) the tracheostomy incision having been placed too inferior in the neck; (2) an artery that is aberrant or abnormally high; (3) an excessively long or poorly fitting tube, which may erode through the anterior wall of the trachea and erode the artery; (4) an overinflated cuff, which may cause ischemic necrosis of the trachea; and (5) tracheal infection, which erodes through the trachea into the innominate artery.

Erosion of the innominate artery is usually preceded by the "sentinel bleed," during which the patient coughs up a small amount of bright red blood prior to the actual massive hemorrhage. All patients with more than minimal tracheal bleeding should be brought to the operating room immediately for bronchoscopy and evaluation. When a tracheoinnominate fistula is recognized, a cuffed tube should be inserted into the trachea, the cuff maximally inflated, and suprasternal pressure applied. Blood for transfusion should be available during transport to the operating room, where sternotomy and control of the innominate artery is performed.[25] The survival rate without these maneuvers is only 7%, but survival increases to 50% if the problem is recognized and treated in a timely way by these maneuvers.[26] Therefore, a high index of suspicion is necessary when any bleeding occurs in a patient with a tracheostomy.

Persistent Tracheocutaneous Fistula

Following decannulation, a tracheostomy tract that is lined with mature squamous epithelium may not close spontaneously. A tract associated with a small scar may be treated surgically by simply excising the epithelial tract and allowing the wound to close. If the tract is associated with a large, depressed cosmetically unacceptable scar, the scar and tract should be excised but the wound closed loosely and a Penrose drain placed, leaving an opening in the skin over the tracheostomy for air to escape. This method prevents potential air dissection, which frequently occurs when the wound is closed tightly. The scar that is left following healing is quite acceptable. Overnight hospital observation is recommended following closure of tracheocutaneous fistulae to observe for air dissection. Persistent tracheocutaneous fistulae occur commonly follow the "starplasty" type tracheostomy.[7]

SUMMARY

Preoperative planning is the first step for successful tracheostomy in the pediatric population. This includes a thorough case history, physical examination, and excellent communication between anesthesiologist and surgeon. Trained personnel in the operating room, emergency room, or intensive care unit must be available to provide the appropriate support during and after the surgical procedure. Postoperative care should extend for at least 5 days in the intensive care unit, at which time the stoma is healed, and the first tube change is generally performed. All members of the team should be aware of the major signs that signal a complication. Despite proper timing and performance of this operation under optimum circumstances, complications may occur. Intraoperative, postoperative, and late complications of tracheostomy may be severe; however, when the proper steps are taken at each phase, complications may be minimized and their proper treatment will reduce the likelihood of a catastrophic outcome.

REFERENCES

1. Lewis CW, Carron JD, Perkins JA, Sie KCY, Feudtner C. Tracheostomy in pediatric patients: a national perspective. *Arch Otolaryngol Head Neck Surg.* 2003;129(5):523-529.

2. Hartnick J, Bissell C, Parsons SK. The impact of pediatric tracheostomy on parental caregiver burden and health status. *Arch Otolaryngol Head Neck Surg.* 2003;129(10):1065-1069.

3. Tantinikorn W, Alper CM, Bluestone CD, Casselbrant ML. Outcome in pediatric tracheostomy. *Am J Otolaryngol.* 2003; 24(3):131-137.

4. Rabuzzi DD, Reed GF. Intrathoracic complications following tracheostomy in children. *Laryngoscope.* 1971;81(6):939-946.

5. Parnes SM, Myers EN. Traction sutures in a tracheostomy using a ligature passer. *Trans Sect Otolaryngol Am Acad Opthalmol Otolaryngol.* 1976;82(4):479-485.

6. Solares CA, Krakovitz P, Hirose K, Koltai PJ. Starplasty: revisiting a pediatric tracheostomy technique. *Otolaryngol Head Neck Surg.* 2004;131(5):717-722.

7. Sautter NB, Krakovitz PR, Solares CA, Koltai PJ. Closure of persistent tracheocutaneous fistula following "starplasty" tracheostomy in children. *Int J Pediatr Otorhinolaryngol.* 2006;70(1):99-105.

8. Greenberg JS, Sulek M, de Jong A, Friedman EM. The role of postoperative chest radiography in pediatric tracheostomy. *Int J Pediatr Otorhinolaryngol.* 2001; 60(1):41-47.

9. Pinto JM, Ansley J, Baroody FM. Lack of utility of postoperative chest radiograph in pediatric tracheostomy. *Otolaryngol Head Neck Surg.* 2001;125(3):241-244.

10. Ruben RJ, Newton L, Jornsay D, et al. Home care of the patient with a tracheostomy. *Ann Otol Rhinol Laryngol.* 1982;91(6 pt 1):633-640.

11. Greene NM, Fatal cardiovascular and respiratory failure associated with tracheostomy. *N Engl J Med.* 1959;261:846-848.

12. Galvis AG, Stool SE, Bluestone CD. Pulmonary edema following relief of acute upper airway obstruction. *Ann Otol Rhinol Laryngol.* 1980;89(2 pt 1): 124-128.

13. Morar P, Singh V, Makura Z, et al. Oropharyngeal carriage and lower airway colonization/infection in 45 tracheotomised children. *Thorax.* 2002;57(12):1015-1020.

14. Perkins J, Mouzakes J, Pereira R, Manning S. Bacterial biofilm presence in pediatric tracheostomy tubes. *Arch Otolaryngol Head Neck Surg.* 2004;130(3):339-343.

15. Sasaki CT, Suzuki M, Horiuchi M, Kirchner JA. The effect of tracheostomy on the laryngeal closure reflex. *Laryngoscope.* 1977;87(9 pt 1):1428-1433.

16. Finder JD, Yellon RF, Charron M. Successful management of tracheotomized patients with chronic saliva aspiration by use of constant positive airway pressure. *Pediatrics.* 2001;107(6):1343-1345.

17. Yellon RF. Totally obstructing tracheostomy-associated suprastomal granulation tissue. *Int J Pediatr Otorhinolaryngol.* 2000; 53(1):49-55.

18. Gupta A, Cotton RT, Rutter MJ. Pediatric suprastomal granuloma: management and treatment. *Otolaryngol Head Neck Surg.* 2004;131(1):21-25.

19. Rimell FL, Shapiro AM, Mitskavich MT, Modreck P, Post JC, Maisel RH. Pediatric fiberoptic laser rigid bronchoscopy. *Otolaryngol Head Neck Surg.* 1996;114(3): 413-417.

20. Rosenfeld RM, Stool SE. Should granulomas be excised in children with long-term tracheostomy? *Arch Otolaryngol Head Neck Surg.* 1992;118(12):1323-1327.

21. Mandell DL, Yellon RF. Endoscopic KTP laser excision of severe tracheostomy-associated suprastomal collapse. *Int J Pediatr Otorhinolaryngol.* 2004;68: 1423-1428.

22. Borowiecki B, Croft BE. Experimental model of subglottic stenosis. *Ann Otol Rhinol Laryngol.* 1977;86(6 pt 1):835-840.

23. Sasaki CT, Horiuchi M, Koss N. Tracheostomy related subglottic stenosis:

bacteriologic pathogenesis. *Laryngoscope.* 1979;89:857–865.

24. Little FB, Koufman JA, Kohut RI, Marshall RB. Effect of gastric acid on the pathogenesis of subglottic stenosis. *Ann Otol Rhinol Laryngol.* 1985;94(5 pt 1):516–519.

25. Bloss RS, Ward RE. Survival after tracheoinnominate artery fistula. *Am J Surg.* 1980;139(2):251–253.

26. Jones JW, Reynolds M, Hewitt RL, Drapanas T. Tracheoinnominate artery erosion: successful surgical management of a devastating complication. *Ann Surg.* 1976;184(2):194–204.

CHAPTER 5

Tracheostomy in the Intensive Care Unit Setting

KAREN M. KOST

Critically ill patients represent a particular subset of the population by virtue of their multisystem disease and the complexity of the care they require. Tracheostomy is a frequently performed procedure in this patient population and requires special consideration in terms of indications, technique, and care. Endoscopic percutaneous tracheostomy is especially well suited to patients in the intensive care unit (ICU) and, as such, is discussed in a comprehensive fashion. Special attention is also given to tracheostomy care-related issues such as: cuff pressure, cleaning and suctioning, infection, communication, and feeding.

PERCUTANEOUS TRACHEOSTOMY

Our ability to keep critically ill patients alive on mechanical ventilation has improved dramatically over the past 60 years. Paralleling this trend has been the increased need for tracheostomy. As a result, now more than half of the tracheostomies today are performed on intubated patients in the ICU.[1] These patients frequently have multiorgan diseases and, as such, are at higher risk for complications than other groups. Stauffer et al[2] noted a 66% complication rate in tracheotomies performed on patients in the ICU; Zeitouni and Kost[1] noted a 30% complication rate in patients in the ICU undergoing tracheostomy compared to a 17% rate in patients outside the ICU.

Traditionally these patients have been taken to the operating room (OR) for a "standard" tracheostomy (ST), which is usually a variation of Chevalier Jackson's technique using sharp dissection. With few exceptions, these patients are already intubated and the procedure is considered semielective; therefore, they are given a low OR priority. OR time is expensive, in high demand, and often in short supply. Consequently the procedure may be performed late at night one or more days after the initial consultation. Moving these critically ill patients with their monitors requires additional personnel and carries a number of different risks, including accidental extubation and vital sign changes requiring pharmacologic intervention.[3-6] These factors have led to an interest in developing a safe, convenient, and cost-effective procedure that can be performed at the bedside.

Standard tracheostomy at the bedside is often inconvenient and requires transporting instrument trays, adequate suction, extra lighting, and electrocautery from the OR. The procedure may be further compromised by the lack of trained OR nurses and assistants. Risks include inadequate or difficult visualization, and spontaneous ignition with the use of electrocautery in the presence of $\geq 30\%$ O_2.

Seldinger's[7] description in 1953 of catheter replacement of the needle in percutaneous anteriography over a guidewire served as a basis for the development of several percutaneous tracheostomy techniques.[8-10] Although many of these early procedures were quickly abandoned, interest in this area persisted, and

in 1985, when Ciaglia[11] described bedside percutaneous dilatational tracheostomy, the procedure was rapidly adopted in many ICUs, principally by critical care physicians and anaesthesiologists. The technique is based on progressive dilatation of an initial tracheal puncture and has been recommended particularly for patients in the ICU. There were early concerns over safety because the procedure, as originally described, is blind.[12] With the notable addition of endoscopic guidance, first reported in 61 patients by Marelli et al,[13] the "blind aspect" has been addressed. This author's experience with over 500 cases to date has demonstrated that, with bronchoscopic visualization and attention to technical detail, endoscopic percutaneous dilatational tracheostomy (PDT) is a safe, cost-effective alternative to ST in the OR, to complication rates comparable to or lower than those of ST.

Patient Selection

It must be stressed that PDT is suitable only in adult intubated patients (Table 5-1). This patient population accounts for almost two-thirds of all tracheostomies performed today.[1] The more common indications include:

1. Removing the endotracheal tube
2. Aid in weaning from mechanical respiration
3. Pulmonary toilet
4. Upper airway obstruction.

Anatomic and medical suitability for this procedure must be determined preoperatively with the patient's neck extended.[14,15] Contraindications to the procedure (see Table 5-1) include the

Table 5–1. Indications and Contraindications for Percutaneous Tracheostomy

Indications
• Adult intubated ICU patients
Contraindications
• Inability to palpate the cricoid cartilage
• Midline neck mass
• High innominate artery
• Unprotected airway
• Emergencies
• Children
• PEEP ≥15 cm H_2O
• Uncorrected coagulopathy (relative contraindication)

inability to palpate the cricoid cartilage above the sternal notch, the presence of a midline neck mass, a high innominate artery, or large thyroid gland. Patients with these conditions should undergo ST in the OR. Coagulopathies are common in this patient population and should be corrected as much as the patient's condition allows preoperatively. Ideally, platelets should be ≥50,000 and the International Normalized Ratio (INR) corrected to ≤1.5. Patients requiring a positive end-expiratory pressure (PEEP) of ≥15 cm H_2O are at high risk for complications such as subcutaneous emphysema and pneumothorax and should undergo ST in the OR.

Nonintubated patients with acute airway compromise constitute an absolute contraindication to PCT. The procedure requires a secure airway for bronchoscopic visualization through an endotracheal (ET) tube or laryngeal mask airway. The different airway anatomy and dimensions in the pediatric population as well as the technical difficulties of maintaining adequate ventilation with a bronchoscope within a small ET tube renders the procedure completely unsuitable in this age group (see Table 5-1).

Preoperative Planning

Preoperative testing is minimal and includes a recent chest radiograph as well as serum determination of hemoglobin, prothrombin time, partial thromboplastin time, and platelets. Cross-matching is not necessary even in the presence of low hemoglobin levels. A fully equipped intubation cart should be available nearby in the event of accidental extubation during the procedure. Special consideration should be given to obese patients or those with a short, thick neck. Thick subcutaneous tissues in this group place them at particular risk for accidental decannulation. This potential problem may be circumvented by using an extended length (proximal) tracheostomy tube.[14]

Personnel

Four people are required, including the attending staff surgeon, a resident or critical care colleague to perform the bronchoscopy, and a respiratory technician to assist in suctioning, adjusting ventilator settings, and holding the ET tube firmly in position. A nurse is needed to administer medication, monitor vital signs, and help in obtaining necessary materials and instruments. The surgeon and necessary instruments are positioned to the patient's right, the respiratory technician to the left, and the bronchoscopist at the head of the bed.

Instruments

At present two kits are commercially available for this procedure, and both are designed for single use. The first of these, the Ciaglia Percutaneous Tracheostomy Introducer Kit (Cook Critical Care Inc., Bloomington, Ind), relies on eight curved graduated dilators (from 12 to 38 French) for progressive dilatation of an initial tracheal puncture. The procedure was simplified in 1998 with the introduction of the Ciaglia Blue Rhino Percutaneous Introducer Kit (Cook Critical Care Inc., Bloomington, Ind) which allows for dilatation using a single, sharply tapered dilator with a hydrophilic coating. With both kits, the tracheostomy tube is fitted with a loading dilator prior to insertion. A 26-French loading dilator is required to insert a No. 6 Shiley tracheostomy tube, whereas a 28-French loading dilator is used to insert a No. 8 Shiley tracheostomy tube. Shiley "Per-Fit" tracheostomy tubes are commercially available and have been specially designed and tapered to permit for easier insertion. The size of the tube can be determined at the time of the procedure.

Other required instruments include a scalpel, curved hemostat, straight scissors, a needle driver, nonresorbable sutures, water-based lubricant, two 10-mL syringes, and an appropriately sized tracheostomy tube. The instruments should be placed on an instrument stand over the patient's bed and in the order in which they are to be used. An appropriately sized bronchoscope with a suction port must be chosen to fit within the ET tube while still allowing adequate ventilation. A pediatric bronchoscope may be required for ET tubes less than 8 mm. Almost any bronchoscope may be used in patients ventilated through a laryngeal mask airway. A video monitor, if available, may be connected to the bronchoscope, allowing full visualization of the intratracheal portion of the procedure by the operating surgeon and staff.

Anesthesia

Any procedure involving manipulation of the trachea is highly stimulating to the patient and requires adequate local anesthesia supplemented by intravenous sedation. Local anesthesia, consisting of 1% or 2% lidocaine with 1:100,000 epinephrine is used for generous infiltration of the incision site and pretracheal soft tissue. Topical anesthesia in the form of 2% to 4% lidocaine may be injected through the bronchoscope and is useful in decreasing the cough reflex. Intravenous sedation is also required with the particular drug combination dependent on the individual patient and the institution. Frequently used medications include propofol, administered as a continuous infusion or in boluses, midazolam, and sublimaze (Fentanyl). Muscle relaxants such as pancuronium bromide may be used as an adjunct in cases where agitation is a problem. The presence of an anesthetist is optional and may depend on hospital policy. Care should be exercised in administering these medications particularly in the elderly as large fluctuations in blood pressure and heart rate may occur even with small doses.

Technique

Following appropriate sedation, ventilator settings are adjusted to deliver 100% O_2 and allow for the presence of the bronchoscope. Vital signs including heart rate, blood pressure, and oxygen saturation are monitored continuously throughout the procedure. The instruments for the Ciaglia Blue Rhino Introducer Set are illustrated in Figure 5–1. Instruments are laid out on a Mayo stand in the anticipated order of use (Fig 5–2). The patient is positioned as for conventional tracheostomy with the neck extended provided that there is no contraindication (eg, cervical spine fracture). Important anatomic landmarks including the thyroid and cricoid cartilages, and sternal notch are palpated. The patient's neck and upper chest are then prepped and draped in a standard fashion and the incision site is infiltrated with 2% lidocaine with 1:100,000 epinephrine.

A 1.5- to 2-cm skin incision, just long enough to insert a tracheostomy tube, is made at the level of the first and second tracheal rings. This corresponds to approximately one fingerbreadth above the sternal notch or two fingerbreadths below

the cricoid. The subcutaneous tissues are gently separated horizontally with a curved hemostat to allow accurate palpation of the cricoid cartilage and tracheal rings. No attempt is made to divide or otherwise manipulate the isthmus of the thyroid gland.

At this point the patient is suctioned and 1 to 2 mL of 4% lidocaine may be instilled into the ET tube to decrease coughing. Any tapes or ties must be loosened to allow manipulation of the ET tube. An appropriately sized flexible bronchoscope with a suction port is inserted through an adapter into the ET tube and advanced until the tip of the bronchoscope lies flush with the ET tube. During this step, the bronchoscope light will be seen through the incision as it is advanced into the ET tube. From this point on, the ET tube must be held securely by the bronchoscopist or respiratory technician to prevent accidental extubation. The ET tube (with the cuff

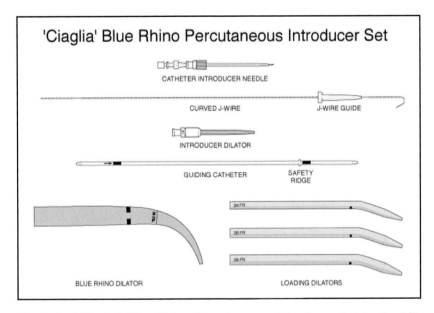

Fig 5–1. "Ciaglia" Blue Rhino Percutaneous Introducer Set by Cook™. Instruments in the single dilator kit.

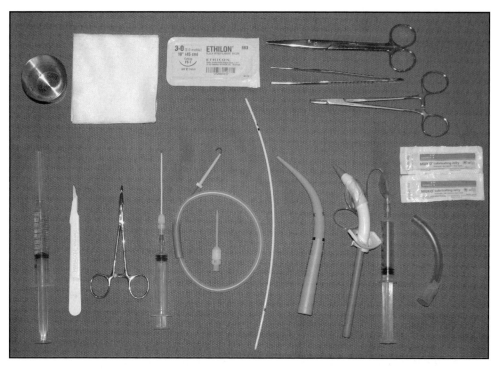

Fig 5–2. Cook™ kit: Instruments arranged in order of use. *Left to right*: (1) Syringe with local anaesthesia (2) Scalpel (3) Hemostat (4) Syringe with 16-gauge introducer needle (5) J-wire (6) 14 French introducer dilator (7) Guiding catheter (8) Single dilator (9) Tracheostomy tube. *Top*: saline to activate the hydrophilic coating, gauze, silk suture, straight scissors, toothed forceps, needle driver.

momentarily deflated) and bronchoscope are slowly withdrawn as a unit until the incision is transilluminated and/or digital depression of the trachea is endoscopically visualized. All ensuing steps are visualized through the bronchoscope. With the ET tube and bronchoscope properly positioned, the tracheal rings are palpated and a No. 14 or No. 16 Teflon catheter introducer needle is inserted between the first and second or second and third tracheal rings (Fig 5-3). The location of the needle is verified endoscopically and modified until a midline intercartilaginous position is achieved. Care is taken not to puncture the posterior tracheal wall. The needle is removed

and a J-tipped guidewire is threaded through the remaining catheter into the trachea (Fig 5-4). This catheter sheath is removed and replaced by a 14-French introducer dilator (Fig 5-5). Removal of this introducer dilator facilitates the passage and positioning of the 12-French guiding catheter over the guidewire between the markings. The guiding catheter and J-wire then form a unit (Fig 5-6) over which further dilatations are achieved. Until 1998, subsequent dilatation was achieved by using a series of eight progressively larger dilators. Since that time, dilatation is more easily accomplished using a single, sharply tapered soft-tipped dilator with a hydrophilic

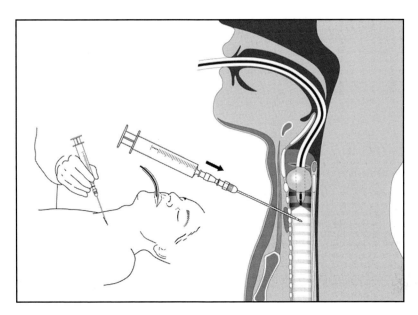

Fig 5–3. With the bronchoscope positioned within the endotracheal tube, the 16-gauge introducer needle is inserted between the first and second or second and third tracheal rings. Note position of endotracheal tube with the cuff just below the vocal folds. The bronchoscope projects a short distance beyond the tip of the ET tube.

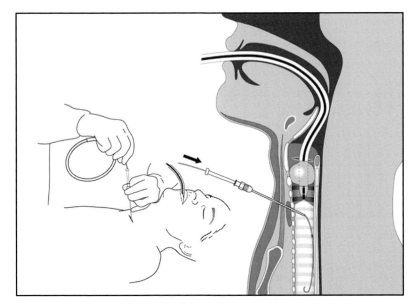

Fig 5–4. The 16-gauge introducer needle is removed, leaving only the sheath, through which the J-tipped guidewire is introduced.

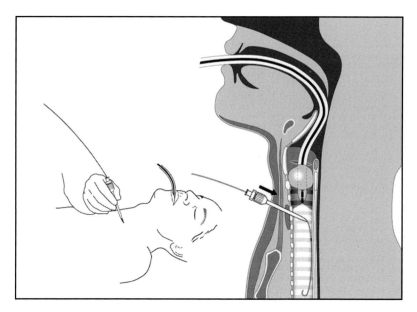

Fig 5–5. The introducer needle Teflon sheath is removed and replaced by the 14-French introducer dilator. This facilitates the next step, placement of the 12-French guiding catheter.

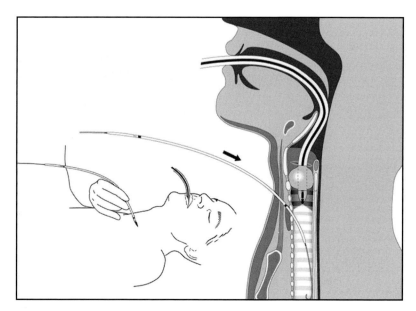

Fig 5–6. The 14-French introducer dilator is removed, and replaced by the 12-French guiding catheter which is positioned over the guide-wire between the markings. Note the direction of the arrow and the small ridge (placed close to the skin) on the guiding catheter. The J-wire guiding catheter unit forms a unit over which subsequent dilatation is achieved.

coating activated by dipping it in saline. This single dilator is held like a pen, and introduced over the guidewire/guiding catheter unit in an arc conforming to the tract undergoing dilatation. Some collapse of the anterior tracheal wall may occur during dilatation (Fig 5–7). Slight overdilatation facilitates placement of the tracheostomy tube. The tracheostomy tube, prefitted with the appropriately sized loading dilator, is threaded over the guidewire/guiding catheter unit into the trachea (Fig 5–8). Two points of resistance typically are encountered during this maneuvre: the interface between the loading dilator and tracheostomy tube, and upon insertion of the balloon.

At this point, the dilator, guiding catheter, and J-wire are removed (Fig 5–9) and replaced with the inner cannula. The cuff is inflated and ventilation is continued through the tracheostomy tube. The tracheostomy tube is secured with four corner sutures and tape ties. Blood and/or secretions are suctioned from the trachea. Only when adequate ventilation is established can the ET tube be removed. The vocal cords may be inspected upon removal of the bronchoscope and ET tube.

Tracheostomy tube size is chosen based on the clinical needs and gender of the patient with a preference for smaller No. 6 internal diameter (I.D.) tubes in females whenever possible. In a patient with a short, thick neck, a longer tracheostomy tube should be used to prevent accidental displacement of the tube into the pretracheal soft tissue.

Depending on the degree of calcification of the tracheal cartilages, fracture of the ring immediately adjacent to the

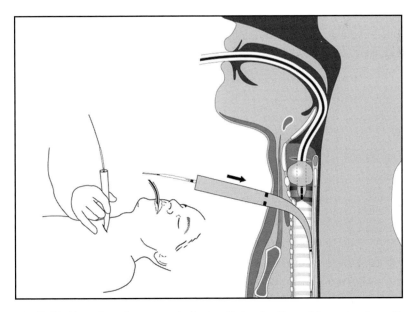

Fig 5–7. The sharply tapered single dilator is dipped in water to activate its hydrophilic coating. It is held like a pen and introduced over the J-wire/guiding catheter unit into the trachea. Slight overdilatation is desirable to facilitate placement of the tracheostomy tube.

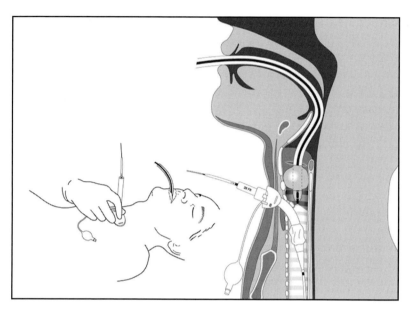

Fig 5–8. The tracheostomy tube, prefitted with the appropriate loading dilator, is advanced over the J-wire/guiding catheter unit into the trachea.

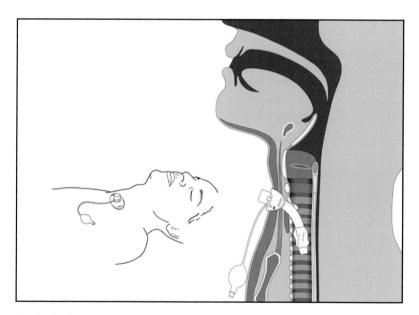

Fig 5–9. The loading dilator, J-wire, and guiding catheter are removed and replaced by the inner cannula.

dilator may occur during dilatation. This is akin to intentionally incising one (or more) ring during an open surgical tracheostomy. This is clinically insignificant and does not increase the incidence of trachomalacia and tracheal stenosis.[14]

Postoperative Considerations

Particular care is taken in monitoring for changes in vital signs such as hypotension, tachycardia, or O_2 desaturation. With the termination of the intense stimulation produced by the procedure, the effects of the sedation may become more pronounced, resulting in hypotension and requiring pharmacologic correction. Suctioning may be required to clear secretions or blood thus preventing a drop in O_2 saturation. A postoperative chest radiograph is required to ensure the absence of pneumothorax and pneumomediastinum.

Many of these patients have copious secretions from the tracheostomy site from their associated pulmonary condition. A tracheostomy tube with an inner cannula facilitates care and hygiene and ensures added safety by allowing rapid removal should obstruction from secretions occur. The PDT technique is primarily dilatational with minimal tissue dissection resulting in a tighter tract and a very snug fit of the tracheostomy tube. The technique does not allow placement of traction sutures at the level of the trachea. Because of these factors, the patient should be reintubated orally in the event of accidental decannulation within the first 7 days of the procedure while the tract is still relatively immature. Although not specifically reported, attempts at replacing the tracheostomy tube in an emergency situation could result in bleeding, the creation of a false passage (Fig 5–10), pneumomediastinum, hypoxia, and even death.

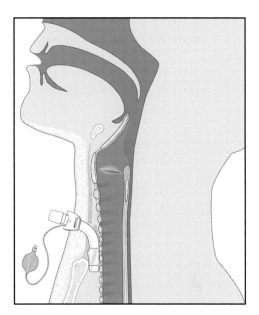

Fig 5–10. Displacement of tracheostomy tube out of the trachea and into the soft tissues in a patient with exceptionally thick pretracheal tissues. Extended length tracheostomy tubes should be used in these situations.

Table 5–2. Intraoperative Complications of Percutaneous Tracheostomy

- Desaturation
- Bleeding
- Accidental extubation
- Injury to posterior wall of the trachea
- Technical misadventure
- Pneumothorax
- Pneumomediastinum
- False passage

Complications

Potential intraoperative and postoperative complications are listed in Tables 5-2 and 5-3, respectively. The overall complication rate for endoscopic PDT reported in the literature is 8.3% (853 cases) and 9.2% in the author's series of 500 cases.[14]

These complication rates compare favorably to those of ICU patients undergoing open surgical tracheostomy in the operating room, where complication rates of 14 to 66% have been reported,[1,2,16,17-19] or at the bedside where complication rates of 4 to 41% have been reported.[20-25] Although it has been argued that endoscopic visualization may not be necessary to safely perform PDT, the literature indicates otherwise (Table 5-4).[14,26-30] The overall complication rate for PDT

performed without endoscopy is 16.8% (1,385 cases), compared to 8.3% (851) in endoscopic PDT, a difference which is highly statistically significant ($p < .0001$).[14]

In the author's series of 500 cases, a significant association (p value $< .05$) was found between body mass index (BMI) = 30 and risk of complications. Fully 15% of patients with a BMI = 30 experienced a complication compared to 8% of patients with a BMI < 30. When "degree of illness," as assessed by the American Society of Anesthesia (ASA) is taken into consideration (Table 5-5), this risk is even more significant. For the subset of patients with a BMI = 30 who were also in ASA class 4, a complication rate of 20% was noted ($p < .02$).[14] The most common complication in this group was accidental decannulation owing to the thickness of the subcutaneous tissues. Use of a proximally extended cannula circumvents this problem. Although it is often stated that obesity is a contraindication

Table 5–3. Postoperative Complications of Percutaneous Tracheostomy

- Bleeding
- Accidental decannulation
- Infection
- Tracheal stenosis
- Tracheomalacia

Table 5–4. Incidence of Serious Complications in Endoscopic versus Nonendoscopic Percutaneous Tracheostomy

Complications	Endoscopic % (N = 851)	Nonendoscopic % (N = 1,385)
# Complications	71/851	233/1,385
% Complications	8.3	16.8

Table 5–5. American Society of Anesthesia Classification

Class 1: healthy patient with no medical problems
Class 2: patient with mild systemic disease
Class 3: patient has severe systemic disease, which is not incapacitating
Class 4: patient has severe systemic disease that is a constant threat to life
Class 5: patient is moribund, not expected to live 24 hours irrespective of operation

to PDT, there are no data to suggest that the risk of complications in obese patients undergoing open surgical tracheostomy is reduced.[14] Similarly, it is often noted that the presence of kyphoscoliosis or a prior tracheostomy constitutes a contraindication to endoscopic PDT. This author's experience[14] indicates that these subsets of patients are not at increased risk of complications.

There is a learning curve for endoscopic PDT, very much in keeping with the learning curves identified in several other minimally invasive techniques.[31,32] In the study involving 500 cases by the current author, a higher rate of complications (40%) is reported in the first 30 patients undergoing endoscopic PDT compared to the remaining 470 patients (9.2%). This difference is statistically significant (*p* <.0001).[14] Appropriate training, careful selection of patients with anatomically favorable necks and cumulative experience reduce the impact and importance of this curve.

Complication rates for surgical and percutaneous tracheotomies, when available, are compared in Table 5-6. This

author's data are amongst the very few available on the risk of tracheostomy in obese patients.

Desaturation

Brief episodes of oxygen desaturation (lasting less than 60 seconds) to below 90%, may occur at the time of tracheostomy tube insertion, particularly in patients with compromised pulmonary function requiring high FiO_2 concentrations.[14] Desaturation is not discussed in the vast majority of articles on either percutaneous or open tracheostomy and the frequency of such events is therefore unknown. In our series, desaturation occurred in 2.8% of the cases.[14] The risk of such an occurrence may be minimized by ventilating all patients on 100% O_2 for the duration of the procedure, and thorough pre/intraoperative suctioning of secretions.

Bleeding

The overall incidence of bleeding for PDT noted in the literature ranges from

Table 5–6. Comparison of Complication Rates for Surgical Versus Percutaneous Tracheotomy

Type of Complication	Surgical (%)	Percutaneous (%)
Mortality	0–2	0–0.5
Accidental decannulation	0–8	0.4–1.4
Bleeding	0–37	1.3–4
Infection	0–19	0.8–1.5
Obesity	N/A	15
Stenosis	0.6–65	2.5

N/A = Not available

1 to 4%, and in most cases is minor.[14] These rates compare favorably with the incidence of bleeding for a standard open tracheostomy, (performed in the ICU or in the operating room), reported to be from 0%[33] to 37%,[2] with most reports falling somewhere in between.[14] Life-threatening hemorrhage is a rare event, and has been noted for both PDT and ST in isolated reports.[34-36] The relatively low incidence of bleeding complications associated with PDT can be explained by the blunt nature of the technique as well as the tamponade effect of the tracheostomy tube against the tight tract which is created.

Infection

Overall infection rates for PDT are reported to be 1.5% (34/2237) whereas infection rates for open surgical tracheostomy, when reported, range from 0% to 19%.[1,2,16,37,38] Because of the small wound and tight tract in PDT, the surface area available for bacterial colonization[26] is markedly reduced compared to that following the sharp, soft tissue dissection in ST.[14,15]

Accidental Extubation

The true incidence of accidental extubation for either PDT or open surgical tracheostomy is difficult to estimate because it is infrequently mentioned in the literature. This complication occurred in three patients early in our series of 500 cases and all were successfully reintubated.[14] The risk of this complication may be reduced through the following steps: the ETT should be held and manipulated only by a physician with the assistance (when needed) of a respiratory therapist and such manipulation should only occur after the bronchoscope has been inserted.

Posterior Wall Injury

Occasional overzealous initial needle insertion may puncture the posterior wall, but this is clinically insignificant and is easily corrected by simply withdrawing the needle to the appropriate position. Serious posterior wall injury is more likely to occur when the procedure is done in a "blind" fashion without bronchoscopy. This complication may be avoided by attention to technical detail (proper positioning of the guidewire, guiding catheter, and dilator) and, most importantly, constant endoscopic visualization of the posterior wall during the procedure.[14]

Technical Misadventures

Loss of the puncture site and accidental removal of the J-wire include some of the possible technical mishaps. In these instances the procedure must be continued from the previous step or started anew as dictated by the circumstances. Occasionally, dilatation may be difficult and undue resistance is encountered. In these cases, the size of the incision and the adequacy of the soft tissue "tunnel" should be verified. Additional spreading of the soft tissue should correct the problem. As a general rule, the surgeon's index finger should fit comfortably in the incision and soft tissue tunnel. If the initial needle insertion is through a tracheal ring, dilatation will be difficult or impossible. The needle must be repositioned such that it enters between rings. If the tracheostomy tube is difficult to insert, the tract should be "re-dilated." The use of excessive force during any step of the procedure always indicates a problem. Excessive force should never be used and is likely to lead to complications and/or damage the instruments. Technical problems may prolong the procedure but rarely directly impact patient safety or outcome.[14]

False Passage, Pneumothorax, and Pneumomediastinum

These potentially fatal complications can be almost completely avoided by continuous bronchoscopic visualization of every step of the procedure. Excessive force should never be used during dilatation or tracheostomy tube insertion, and always indicates a technical problem.

Accidental Decannulation

Accidental decannulation is unusual because of the tight tract. Most at risk are obese patients or those with short, thick necks in whom subcutaneous adipose effectively shortens the intratracheal length of the tracheostomy tube. This potential problem may be circumvented by using proximally extended-length tracheostomy tubes.[14]

Tracheal Stenosis and Tracheomalacia

Attempts to evaluate the incidence of late sequelae for both open surgical and percutaneous tracheostomy are hampered by the high mortality of ICU patients and the difficulty in obtaining long-term follow-up. Compilation of available data reveals a 2.5% incidence of late sequelae in percutaneous tracheostomy[14,20,39–46] compared to a 0.6 to 65% incidence reported for open surgical tracheoto-

mies.[2,33,37,44] Steps toward decreasing the occurrence of these sequelae include: (1) proper placement of the tracheostomy tube between the first and third tracheal rings, (2) use of the smallest possible tube size, (3) minimizing cuff inflation pressures and (4) minimizing cuff inflation times.

Other Considerations

Several studies have documented reduced operative time for PDT compared to surgical tracheostomy.[18,19,25,26,28,48,49] From a training perspective, most residents consider endoscopic PDT to be easier than surgical tracheostomy. Furthermore, Barba et al[28] noted that endoscopic PDT was classified as "easy" by a significantly larger number of surgeons compared with surgical tracheostomy.

The results of several cost analyses have demonstrated a clear cost advantage to PDT when compared with open surgical tracheostomy in the OR.[13,14,28,29,45,47] The cost of PDT is slightly higher when compared to open bedside tracheostomy because of the cost of the kit.[14,25] The simple instrumentation, convenience, and scheduling flexibility of bedside PDT constitute significant advantages which offset minor cost differences. By circumventing the OR, endoscopic PDT significantly reduces interval time from consultation to tracheostomy.[14,19,48] This is in the best interests of the patient and the ICU.

As reflected in the literature, endoscopic PDT is firmly and increasingly embraced by anesthesiologists and critical care physicians as a safe and practical bedside procedure both in Europe and North America. Despite a thorough knowledge of the anatomy of the neck, surgical experience, and airway expertise, relatively few otolaryngologists have adopted the procedure. In some centers, this trend has significantly reduced the head and neck surgeon's involvement and experience in tracheotomies done in the ICU.

Summary

The current literature as well as our evaluation of 500 cases of endoscopic percutaneous dilatational tracheostomies support the procedure as an attractive and safe alternative to open surgical tracheostomy at the bedside in adult intubated ICU patients. Obese individuals are at an increased risk for complications, in particular, accidental decannulation. Extended-length tracheostomy tubes should be used in these patients. There is no evidence at the present time to suggest that open surgical tracheostomy in this patient subset is any safer. As with all minimally invasive procedures, there is a learning curve for endoscopic PCT, which may be minimized by obtaining appropriate training prior to commencing the procedure, and selecting patients with "easy" necks initially. The use of bronchoscopy is strongly associated with a decrease in life-threatening complications such as pneumothorax, pneumomediastinum, false passage, and even death, and its use should be mandatory in all cases.

The weight of the literature now clearly establishes endoscopic PDT as being at least as safe as surgical tracheostomy. Furthermore, it is rapid, simple, convenient, and completely independent of OR schedules. As the airway experts, otolaryngologists have the opportunity to learn and teach this minimally invasive procedure as it should be done.

TRACHEOSTOMY TUBE CHANGES

Most reports and textbooks advocate the first postoperative tracheostomy tube change at 5 to 7 days, or once the tract has matured. The ideal timing for routine tracheostomy tube replacement following this first change, however, has received little attention in the literature. This is partly because the operating surgeon is less involved following the "acute postoperative period," and/or patients are transferred to other facilities. The prolonged presence of the same indwelling tracheostomy tube, which is a foreign body, elicits an inflammatory tissue response favoring the growth of granulation tissue, increased secretions, and bacterial colonization with biofilm production.

Granulation tissue is considered to be a late complication or sequelae of tracheostomy, variably reported as occurring in 0.3 to 80% of cases.[50] The clinical importance of granulation tissue lies in its ability to bleed, complicate tracheostomy tube changes, delay attempts at decannulation, and completely obstruct the tracheostomy tube with potentially catastrophic results. Factors thought to favor formation of granulation tissue include bacterial infection, gastroesophageal reflux, suture material, and powder from surgical gloves. Although a number of topical treatments such as steroid creams, antibiotic ointments, and silver nitrate have been suggested, larger amounts of granulation tissue, particularly when obstructive, may require surgical excision, with or without the use of the laser.

Tracheostomy tubes are subject to colonization by bacteria such as *Staphylo-*

coccus epidermidis, which are embedded in biofilm. The longer the tube is in place, the heavier the load of biofilm. This biofilm functions as a "coat of armour" of sorts, effectively protecting bacteria from local and/or systemic antibiotics.

Recent evidence indicates that regular tracheostomy tube changes every 2 weeks for admitted patients, particularly those who are ventilator-dependent, may decrease the incidence of granulation tissue and biofilm formation.[50] As such, tracheostomy tube changes every 2 weeks in this patient subset should be adopted as routine policy.

CUFF PRESSURES

Tracheostomy tube cuffs have two functions: (1) to create a seal against the tracheal mucosa, thereby minimizing aspiration, and (2) to facilitate positive-pressure ventilation by preventing leakage of air.

As a large majority of critically ill patients on mechanical ventilation require an inflated cuff for prolonged periods of time, an understanding of cuff pressures and their effects on the mucosa of the wall of the trachea is both relevant and important. With the accumulated evidence attesting to the injurious effects of low-volume high-pressure cuffs, there has been a gradual shift in the past three decades toward the use of high-volume low-pressure cuffs with the assumption that the latter are safer and to a great extent problem-free. Although they are indeed safer, these newer cuffs are not problem-free. Inappropriate product choice and use may still result in tracheal complications and long-term sequelae.

Low-Volume High-Pressure Cuffs

Tracheal stenosis from low-volume, high-pressure, low-compliance cuffs was a major complication of tracheostomy during the 1960s. These cuffs may exert pressures as high as 180 to 250 mm Hg on the tracheal mucosa before an effective seal is achieved. In addition, the cuffs are spherical and narrow. These characteristics distort the normal C shape of the trachea and result in asymmetric distribution of high pressure over a small contact area (Fig 5–11). The relatively rigid cartilaginous rings are more susceptible to injury than the more yielding posterior membranous portion of the trachea.[51] Ischemic damage to the tracheal mucosa occurs when the mucosal capillary perfusion pressure of 20 to 30 mm Hg is exceeded for significant periods of time.[52] Within 15 minutes of sustained pressure to the wall of the tracheal above 50 mm Hg, epithelial injury occurs, particularly over cartilage. This is followed by histologic inflam-matory changes within 24 to 48 hours. Superficial tracheitis and mucosal ulceration may be seen after several days, progressing to deep ulceration with exposure of cartilage within 1 week. Finally, chondritis with necrosis of cartilage occurs within 2 to 3 weeks. At this point tracheoinnominate and tracheoesophageal fistula may occur. Alternatively, loss of cartilaginous support and healing with granulation tissue and fibrosis may result in tracheal stenosis or tracheomalacia.

High-Volume Low-Pressure Cuffs

The transition in the 1970s to high-volume low-pressure cuffs decreased the incidence of cuff-related tracheal stenosis by

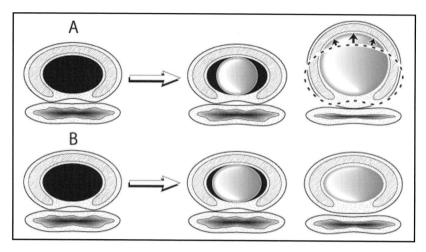

Fig 5–11. Low-volume high-pressure cuffs versus high-volume low-pressure cuffs: effects on tracheal mucosa and shape. **A.** Low-volume high-pressure cuff is short and spherical with a small area of tracheal contact. With inflation the trachea loses its C-shape and assumes the cuff shape. As a result high pressure is asymmetrically distributed to a small contact area. Arrows denote areas of maximum pressure. Capillary perfusion pressure is exceeded, leading to mucosal ischemia, ulceration, and cartilaginous destruction. **B.** High-volume low-pressure cuffs adapt to tracheal contour and allow pressure distribution over a wide area; capillary perfusion pressure is not exceeded.

tenfold[52] because of the ability of the cuff to seal the airway at pressures below mucosal capillary perfusion pressure (Fig 5–12). These cuffs inflate symmetrically, adapt to tracheal contour, and allow pressure distribution over a wide area.

Despite their improved design, these cuffs still have the potential for damaging tracheal mucosa because their pressure-volume characteristics may be altered under different clinical settings and by the relative rigidity within the tracheal wall. In addition, physical characteristics such as cuff length, diameter, thickness, and compliance affect intracuff pressure (Table 5–7). These are discussed below.

Cuff Length

Cuffs of nearly identical diameter but of different lengths provide an equal seal at peak inflation pressures below 25 mm Hg. When lung compliance is reduced and peak inflation pressure is increased, the cuff loses its cylindrical shape and assumes a conical one (Fig 5–13). The shorter cuff, with its relatively small contact area within the tracheal wall, requires a higher cuff pressure to achieve an adequate seal. The cuff then behaves as a high-pressure cuff with the same risks for injury to the wall of the trachea.[51]

Cuff Diameter

Selection of a cuff with the appropriate diameter is also important in preventing injury to the trachea. Cuffs with a diameter smaller than the diameter of the trachea behave as high-pressure cuffs as they must be overinflated, or stretched, to achieve an adequate seal. Cuff diame-

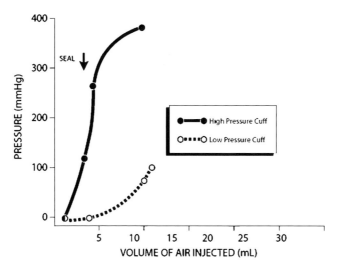

Fig 5–12. Comparison of pressure volume curves of low-volume high-pressure cuffs (*solid line*) and high-volume low-pressure cuffs (*dotted line*). Intracuff pressure in mm Hg is shown on the vertical axis and reflects intratracheal pressure.

Table 5–7. High-Volume Low-Pressure Cuffs: Factors Affecting Cuff Pressures

Cuff Characteristics (endogenous):
1. Cuff length
2. Cuff diameter
3. Cuff thickness
4. Cuff compliance
Clinical settings (exogenous):
1. Increased lung compliance
2. Large trachea

ters vary from 24.7 to 32 mm for tracheostomy tubes from different manufacturers with an inner diameter of 8 mm. The diameter of the human trachea is also quite variable and must be estimated. Cuff diameter should exceed the diameter of the patient's trachea if intracuff pressure is to be low. In males, mean tracheal diameter ±1 SD is 27.1 mm and

an adequate cuff diameter would be ≥28 mm.[53] Unfortunately, the diameter of the trachea cannot be predicted based on height, weight, or age.

Cuff Thickness and Compliance

Thin-walled, large-diameter, high-compliance cuffs tend to "drape" relatively well against the trachea, thus providing a better seal at low cuff pressures and reducing aspiration (Fig 5–14).[53] The "draping" of these cuffs is not perfect, however, and some longitudinal folds may occur, allowing for microaspiration. This is an important consideration as microaspiration is one of the leading causes of ventilator-associated pneumonia. A newly developed low-volume, low-pressure tracheostomy tube (LMA International SA, Henley, UK) has been shown in both in vitro and in vivo studies to significantly decrease the risk of microaspiration while allowing for adequate capillary perfusion

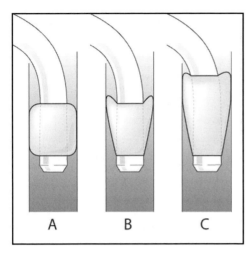

A   B   C

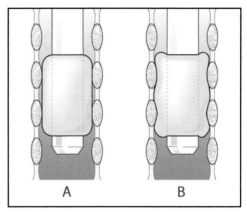

A   B

Fig 5–13. Effect of lung compliance on cuff shape. **A.** Normal lung compliance: the cuff maintains its cylindrical shape, has a wide contact area with the trachea, and behaves, as expected, like a high-volume low-pressure cuff. **B.** Increased lung compliance: the cuff loses its cylindrical shape and assumes a conical one. Because of the small tracheal contact area, a higher cuff pressure is required to achieve an adequate seal. The cuff then behaves as a high-pressure cuff. **C.** Increased lung compliance: using a longer cuff in this setting will still result in a conical shape but the tracheal contact area is increased and a lower cuff pressure is required to maintain an adequate seal.

Fig 5–14. "Draping" characteristics of cuffs. **A.** Thick-walled low-compliance cuff requires higher pressure to provide a good seal. **B.** Ideal cuff: thin walls, large diameter, and high compliance allow the cuff to adapt to tracheal contour. Lower pressures are required to provide a good seal and minimize aspiration.

pressures.[54] Cuff specifications are available from the various manufacturers.

Cuff Inflation

To reduce the risk of high intracuff pressures and consequent injury to the trachea, the minimal-leak inflation technique may be used. During positive-pressure ventilation, the cuff initially is inflated to achieve a total seal; air is removed gradually until a minimal air leak is heard at

peak inspiratory pressure. Ventilator adjustments are then made to compensate for the minimal loss in tidal volume.[51,52]

When a complete seal of the trachea is required to ensure adequate ventilation, a "no leak" technique is recommended. The cuff is inflated initially until there is a minimal leak; at this point, additional air is injected slowly until complete occlusion occurs between the cuff and wall of the trachea.

The risk of overinflation with high intracuff pressures may be minimized by:

1. Having a pressure-controlled cuff with a pressure pop-off valve which prevents inflation beyond 20 mm Hg,
2. Regular measurement of intracuff pressure with a manometer attached to a three- or four-way stopcock; the latter gives more accurate results.

3. Cuff deflation for as long as safely possible in patients who do not require mechanical ventilation.

Special consideration must be given to the patient with an inflated tracheostomy tube cuff who requires general anesthesia. Nitrous oxide rapidly diffuses into cuffs inflated with air, thereby increasing intracuff pressure and volume (Fig 5–15). Herniation of the cuff with airway compromise may result as a consequence of this process (Fig 5–16). Inflating the cuff with anesthetic gas may prevent this complication.

In summary, the thermolabile tracheostomy tube with a large, thin, compliant cuff is least likely to produce damage to the trachea (Table 5–8).

CLEANING AND SUCTIONING

Placement of a tracheostomy tube dramatically alters the normal physiology of the upper airway. Under normal circumstances the nose, principally, along with the upper aerodigestive tract, very efficiently warms, humidifies, and filters inspired air. Dry, cold air is 100% humidified and warmed to 37°C by the time it reaches the lungs. These important functions must be restored artificially in the patient with a tracheostomy to prevent potentially fatal complications.

Humidification of inspired air is critical in all patients receiving short- or long-term ventilation. Dehydration of the respiratory tract results in impaired

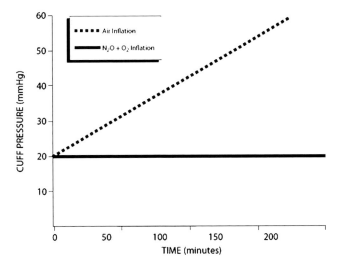

Fig 5–15. Effect of nitrous oxide on intracuff pressure. *Dotted line*: The cuff is inflated with air and nitrous oxide anaesthesia is administered. Nitrous oxide easily diffuses into the cuff during anaesthesia. Cuff pressure and volume increase beyond safe limits thus risking tracheal damage. *Solid line*: Initial cuff inflation with nitrous oxide results in stable cuff pressure and volume during nitrous oxide anaesthesia.

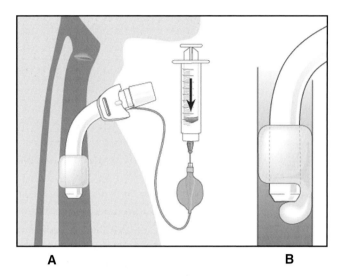

A   **B**

Fig 5–16. Cuff herniation from nitrous oxide anesthesia. **A.** The cuff is inflated with air. Nitrous oxide anesthesia is administered and **B.** diffuses into the cuff; intracuff pressure and volume may increase to the point where cuff herniation occurs, resulting in airway compromise.

Table 5–8. Ideal Characteristics of the High-Volume Low-Pressure Cuff

1. Long cuff
2. Cuff diameter ≥28 mm
3. Thin wall
4. High compliance

mucociliary function, resulting in inspissated secretions and atelectasis. Furthermore, inspiration of dry air may alter pulmonary mechanics by lowering body temperature, increasing pulmonary arteriovenous shunting, and causing bronchoconstriction, thus compromising respiratory function.[55] In patients who do not require mechanical ventilation, humidified air may be delivered through a tracheostomy collar. Hot- and cold-water bedside humidifiers also may be used, with strict attention to careful daily cleaning.[55] Bacterial colonization of the water reservoirs is known to occur and may provide a source of nocosomial infection.

In ventilator-dependent patients, humidification also may be administered through the appropriate tubing. This may be supplemented as needed with nebulized humidification. A heat and moisture exchanger can be used, which works on the principle of returning heat and humidity from the expired gas to the inspired gas.[55]

Production of tenacious secretions is increased following the introduction of a tracheostomy tube. This is a result of irritation of the respiratory mucosa by the tube and the inspiration of dry air. The problem is compounded by impairment of ciliary function and the inability to generate adequate subglottic pressure for an effective cough. Aspiration is associated with tracheostomy to a greater or lesser extent and may contribute to soiling of the tracheobronchial tree even in the presence of an inflated cuff.

Suctioning of secretions to maintain pulmonary toilet and patency of the tracheostomy tube constitutes an integral component of the care of the tracheostomy patient on mechanical ventilation. This, however, should not be carried out as part of a scheduled routine but instead according to the patient's needs. In the early days post-tracheostomy, this may be necessary as frequently as every hour or two. Some patients are able and should be encouraged to cough and clear their airways independently. Indications for suctioning are given in Table 5–9.[56,57]

The seemingly simple procedure of suctioning is not without risk. Hypoxia, cardiac arrhythmia, injury to the tracheobronchial tree, atelectasis, hypoxemia, and infection have all been reported in association with suctioning.[55,56] These events can be minimized by strict attention to technical detail (Table 5–10). Factors that may contribute to hypoxia include the suctioning of oxygen-rich air for too long and the use of inappropriately large catheters. This can be prevented by applying suction for ≤12 seconds with a catheter less than half the size of the tracheostomy tube and ventilating the patient on 100% O_2 for at least five breaths before and after suctioning. Hyperoxygenation has also been shown to prevent cardiac arrhythmias.[55] A strictly aseptic technique while handling the disposable, single-use catheter is mandatory to reduce the risk of cross-contamination.

The catheter should be gently inserted to the level of the carina. A suction pressure of <150 mm Hg is applied only as the catheter is withdrawn.[56] Following these maneuvers minimizes mucosal trauma to the tracheobronchial tree. As an alternative to this open technique, a closed, multiple-use suction catheter, contained within a sheath, may be used. The suctioning technique is the same as for the open system but the catheter requires changing on a daily basis. The closed suction system is associated with a reduced incidence of arterial desaturation during suctioning, possibly owing to the presence of continued mechanical

Table 5–9. Indications for Suctioning

1. Visible secretions in the tracheostomy tube
2. Audible gurgling to the ear or through the stethoscope
3. Coarse or diminished breath sounds
4. Dyspnea
5. Increased airway pressure
6. Unexplained decrease in O_2 saturation levels

Table 5–10. Proper Suctioning Technique

1. Preoxygenate with 100% O_2 for 5 breaths
2. Aseptic technique
3. Use a catheter with less than half the diameter of the tracheostomy tube
4. Insert catheter gently to the carina
5. Suction only on withdrawal
6. Keep suction pressure <150 mm Hg
7. Limit suctioning to 10–12 seconds

ventilation and maintenance of PEEP during the procedure.[58] A further advantage of the system may be a decreased risk of cross-contamination.

Instillation of saline through the tracheostomy tube prior to suctioning is done routinely in many centers to facilitate removal of tenacious secretions. This practice, however, is controversial and has not been shown to be definitively helpful; in fact, it may be associated with some risk. Instilled saline does not reach beyond the trachea and mainstem bronchi; only about 15% is recovered through suctioning, and some studies have demonstrated an adverse effect on oxygen saturation.[55] Cough stimulation, with a resulting loosening of secretions, does occur, but it may be argued that simple insertion of the catheter would produce the same results. Routine instillation of saline is probably not helpful in removing tenacious secretions; if used, it should be restricted to small amounts, such as 2 to 5 mL.

Meticulous care of the tracheostomy tube and peristomal area is important in maintaining a patent airway and preventing infection and breakdown of the skin. Placement of a tracheostomy tube with an inner cannula is mandatory. Soiling of the tracheostomy tube is expected and complete occlusion of the lumen with blood, crusts, secretions, or granulation tissue may occur, resulting in oxygen desaturation, hypoxia, and even death. In this circumstance rapid removal of the inner cannula is potentially life saving. Although continuous humidification is helpful in decreasing the viscosity of secretions, the inner cannula should be removed several times daily in the early postoperative period and thoroughly cleaned in hydrogen peroxide with a soft brush.

Bacterial colonization of the peristomal area is known to occur and cannot be prevented with antibiotics. Attentive wound care with frequent cleaning of accumulated secretions and crusts with hydrogen peroxide will help to prevent breakdown of the skin and the progression from wound colonization to infection. The skin under the tracheostomy neck plate should be kept dry with a thin nonadherent dressing such as Telfa. Petroleum-based products are avoided on open wounds, as they may stimulate granulation tissue and result in myospherulosis. Soiled tracheostomy tapes may cause maceration of the skin and should be replaced as often as necessary. This may be as often as three times daily during the initial postoperative period.

INFECTION

Patients with a tracheostomy tube in place almost invariably have polymicrobial bacterial colonization of the surgical wound as well as the tracheobronchial tree (>80% at 48 hours).[59,60] A number of factors may predispose to this initial colonization and contribute to a possible progression to infection that may include stomatitis, tracheitis, or even pneumonia.

Risk Factors

Disruption of Host Defenses

The skin, which is in itself colonized by relatively harmless bacteria, provides a highly effective natural barrier to infection. Performing a tracheostomy means surgically breaking the integrity of this barrier and, in the case of a standard open tracheostomy, involves a certain amount of sharp dissection to reach the trachea. The resulting incision, which may vary from 3 to 5 cm in length, is left open to prevent subcutaneous emphysema. This open surgical wound provides a wide surface area for colonization, which may occur from surrounding skin, pre-existing infected pulmonary secretions, aspiration of oropharyngeal secretions, instrumentation, or handling of the tracheostomy tube. The integrity of the peristomal skin may be further compromised by prolonged contact with soiled or moist tapes, mechanical pressure, or tension from the neckplate, and by the presence of skin sutures.

Under normal circumstances, natural host defenses against both colonization of the tracheobronchial tree and pulmonary infection begin in the upper airways and include efficient filtration and humidification of air, ciliary transport, and local immunity afforded by Waldeyer's ring. At the level of the larynx, an effective cough reflex and intact mucociliary transport in the tracheobronchial tree provide further protection. In the lung, opsonins, alveolar macrophages, and polymorphonuclear leukocytes provide additional lines of defense.[61]

The patient with a tracheostomy in place does not benefit from most of these protective mechanisms. The nose, paranasal sinuses, and pharynx, where filtration and humidification as well as local leukocyte antibacterial activity occur, are all bypassed. Impaired vocal-fold adduction in patients with tracheostomies, as well as the presence of the tube itself, prevent the generation of an effective cough. The almost universal presence of dysphagia in this patient population further compounds the problem. Copious oropharyngeal secretions,

themselves often colonized with potentially pathogenic gram-negative organisms, are ineffectively cleared or swallowed, allowing some degree of aspiration and contamination of the tracheobronchial tree. The situation is often exacerbated in critically ill patients with impaired consciousness or who are heavily sedated. Mucociliary transport in the trachea and bronchi is compromised by the locally irritative effect of the tracheostomy tube as well as by the inspiration of inadequately humidified air.

Tracheostomy Tube

The majority of tracheostomy tubes and/or cuffs are made of polyvinyl chloride. Of the various plastics used for life support, polyvinyl chloride (PVC) is the one to which bacteria most readily adhere. Polymicrobial flora embedded in a dense polysaccharide biofilm, which is adherent to the surface of the endotracheal tubes, have been demonstrated by electron microscopy.[50,62] This biofilm is present on the majority (>80%) of ET tubes and tracheostomy tubes that have been indwelling for 48 hours or longer. This biofilm may protect bacteria from both antimicrobial and immune defense mechanisms.[62] Adherent microorganisms produce a substance called glycocalyx, a polysaccharide cement that attaches them to each other and to surfaces. Clumps of rod-shaped and coccoid bacteria have been identified within the mass of amorphous matrix (biofilm) projecting from the polyvinyl surfaces of ET and tracheostomy tubes. Cultures of this material have grown a variety of gram-negative and gram-positive bacteria, including *Pseudomonas aeruginosa, Proteus mirabilis, Staphylococcus aureus* and *Staphylococcus epidermidis*—all of which are excellent producers of glycocalyx. These bacterial clumps may then reach the tracheobronchial tree and lungs through detachment and aspiration or be dislodged during suction or bronchoscopy. Tracheostomy tubes that are made of polyvinyl chloride may therefore serve as reservoirs for persistent contamination of the tracheobronchial tree. A recently developed low-volume, low-pressure tracheostomy tube (LMA International SA, Henley, UK) is lined with a "nonstick" surface in an attempt to decrease bacterial adhesion.[54]

Other Bacterial Reservoirs

Medication nebulizers, manual ventilator bags, spirometers, and other respiratory circuit components are all potential sources of respiratory pathogens.[61]

The stomach has received a great deal of attention as a potential bacterial reservoir. Microbial growth in the stomach has been associated with tracheal colonization with the same bacteria, Enterobacteriaceae in particular. These bacteria multiply in situations where gastric acidification is impaired, as with the use of gastric acid-inhibitor therapy.[61] It is uncertain whether these bacteria reach the stomach through retrograde (intestinal tract) or anterograde (mouth) migration. The role of the stomach as a reservoir at this point has not been clearly established.[61]

Infection Sites

Stomal Infection. Colonization of the surgical wound after tracheostomy occurs uniformly, probably within 24 to 48 hours.[59,60] Wound edges may demonstrate mild erythema and secretions (which may be yellow or green) from the area may be copious, particularly in the first 7 to 10 days. These findings are much more marked after standard open tracheostomy than percutaneous tracheostomy, probably because of the very small incision and tight tract in the latter procedure.

Frequent meticulous wound care, with mechanical debridement if necessary, is the best way to deal with this situation. Progressive cellulitis, despite aggressive local care, is an indication for systemic antibiotics. Although cultures should be done prior to initiating treatment, it should be recognized that these infections are usually polymicrobial. Rarely, necrotizing stomal infections may occur, with substantial loss of soft tissue down to and including the tracheal wall. This may create difficulties in maintaining adequate mechanical ventilation. Progression of the process may result in carotid artery exposure, with its attendant risks. Management involves removing the tracheostomy tube, which may be behaving like a foreign body, and replacing it with an ET tube. Aggressive wound debridement and cleaning with antiseptic dressings such as Dakin's 1:64 are also required.[63] Rarely, local flaps may be necessary to provide soft tissue coverage to vital structures.

Tracheitis. Within 48 hours of tracheostomy, up to 80% of patients demonstrate colonization with primarily gram-negative organisms including *Klebsiella, P. aeruginosa,* and *E. coli.*[59] The most common gram-positive isolated is *S. aureus.* This fact, along with mechanical irritation from the tube, cuff, and tube tip means that there is always some degree of localized reversible tracheitis that is often manifest by increased secretions. Progression of this situation may lead to loss of tracheal support, resulting in tracheal stenosis or tracheomalacia. Full-thickness loss may result in life-threatening complications such as tracheoesophageal or tracheoinnominate fistula. Mechanical irritation can be minimized by selecting appropriate tube size, material, and cuff. The cuff should be inflated only when necessary.

The known bacterial colonization of polyvinyl chloride devices makes a strong argument in favor of more frequent tube changes, perhaps weekly, in ventilator-dependent, critically ill patients.

Nosocomial Pneumonia. The most important risk factor in the development of nosocomial pneumonia is the presence of a tracheostomy tube and a colonized trachea as well as mechanical ventilation.[58] Nosocomial pneumonia will occur in 9 to 21% of patients in this subset.[54,60]

Isolated organisms resemble those found in the colonized trachea and include *P. aeruginosa, S. aureus, Klebsiella pneumoniae, E. coli*, and *Enterobacter* species (Table 5–11).[61,64,65] Up to 40% of infections are polymicrobial. Distinguishing between colonization and development of pneumonia may be difficult, as

Table 5–11. Organisms in ICU Patients with Pneumonia

Actinobacter spp
Pseudomonas spp
Staphylococcus aureus
Klebsiella spp
Proteus spp
Escherichia coli
Serratia

fever, leukocytosis, purulent secretions, and pulmonary infiltrates are all common nonspecific findings in the ICU population. Quantitative cultures of the lower airways obtained bronchoscopically using a protected specimen brush and bronchoalveolar lavage techniques may increase accuracy in diagnosing nosocomial pneumonia. This is important, as mortality with this disease is estimated to be as high as 30%.[60,61]

FEEDING

The importance of aggressive nutritional support in the critically ill patient is well recognized. Using bedside examination techniques augmented by modified barium swallows with videofluoroscopy it has been found that among patients requiring mechanical ventilation with tracheostomies in place, the incidence of swallowing dysfunction approaches 80%.[66] The etiology in most cases is multifactorial and may include the following:

1. Glottic injury from previous oro- and/or nasotracheal intubation
2. Limitation of normal laryngeal excursion by the tethering effect of the tracheostomy tube
3. Compression of the esophagus, particularly in the presence of an inflated cuff
4. Desensitization of the larynx and loss of protective reflexes due to chronic air diversion of air through the tube
5. Impaired vocal-fold adduction
6. The use of anxiolytics and/or neuromuscular blocking agents
7. Altered mental status or underlying neuromuscular illness.

For patients on ventilators with minimal swallowing abnormalities and negligible aspiration, oral feedings may be possible, particularly with the help of the speech-language pathologist. Selection of appropriate food consistencies and emphasis on specific head positions may minimize or prevent aspiration. A coached cough reflex and swallowing sequence may also improve swallowing function. In the presence of mild or moderate aspiration, eligible patients on or off the ventilator may benefit from the use of a Passy-Muir valve. This device may reduce aspiration and improve deglutition by restoring subglottic air pressure (see Chapter 3, Technique and Complications of Tracheostomy in Adults).

Unfortunately, for the majority of ventilator-dependent patients with a tracheostomy the degree of swallowing dysfunction is such that oral intake is not an option. Nevertheless, enteral feedings are preferred when the gastrointestinal (GI) tract can be used safely because it is convenient, there are fewer metabolic and infectious complications, and the cost is lower than that of parenteral nutrition.[67] In addition, enterally delivered nutrients are better utilized and provide cytoprotection for the gut mucosa.[68]

Feedings may be provided through small-bore weighted nasoduodenal or nasogastric tubes such as the Dobbhoff tube. It has been proposed that enteral feeding through a nasogastric tube may be associated with an increased risk of gastroesophageal reflux, aspiration, and gastric colonization with gram-negative bacilli by increasing the gastric pH to 6 to 8. By extension, the risk of infection and particularly nosocomial pneumonia may be increased as well. By comparison, jejunal tube feedings may be associated with a lower gastric pH, less gastro-

esophageal reflux, and a reduced risk of aspiration. Attempts to document these differences and ascribe advantages to one method over another have yielded conflicting results and the controversy remains unresolved.[67,69] Both jejunal and gastric feeding tubes can play a role in the nutritional management of critically ill ventilated patients provided that they are used in the appropriate clinical setting.

Nasoduodenal and/or jejunal tubes may be placed in a variety of ways. The simplest of these involves inserting a lubricated small-bore tube with a weighted tip through the nose to a distance of 76 cm. In an effort to stimulate peristalsis and promote transpyloric passage, the patient is then positioned on the right and given drugs such as metoclopropamide. Abdominal roentgenograms are then obtained immediately after insertion and then again after 72 hours to verify tube position. Although this procedure is highly successful in ambulatory patients, it has met with a varying success rate of 15 to 60% in critically ill, ventilated patients.[67,70] Endoscopic placement of jejunal feeding tubes is highly successful but is more costly and carries the inherent risk of gastroscopy. Fluoroscopic placement using a C-arm is also reliable but costly. With all these techniques, dislodgment is still possible; more secure and long-term placement of a postpyloric tube may be achieved using percutaneous endoscopic gastrojejunostomy.

Nasogastric placement of small-bore weighted tubes may also be appropriate in selected patients. Proper positioning of the tube is verified both clinically and by abdominal roentgenogram. Requisites for this type of tube include a functioning GI tract, the presence of intestinal sounds, and the absence of abdominal distention. To minimize complications, aspiration in particular, the head of the bed should be elevated 30 to 40 degrees. Gastric residuals should be verified routinely; if they are greater than 100 mL, tube feedings should be discontinued for 4 hours. The presence or development of abdominal distention also necessitates an interruption in feedings.

For patients with nasogastric or nasojejunal tubes, feedings are begun slowly at 25 mL per hour and gradually increased as tolerated until daily caloric requirements are met. This may take from 3 to 5 days. Feedings should be interrupted if vomiting, diarrhea, abdominal pain, or distention occur. Clinical situations requiring the patient to lie in a flat or Trendelenburg position also warrant interruption of feeding because of the increased risk of aspiration. Percutaneous endoscopic gastrostomy should be considered in patients requiring long-term nutritional support. Examples include patients with severe neurologic impairment and chronic degenerative neuromuscular disorders. Decisions regarding the choice of nutritional support must be individualized in every case to provide maximum benefit and minimal risk to the patient.

INTENSIVE CARE TRACHEOSTOMY TEAM

The principal members of the intensive care tracheostomy team include the surgeon, respiratory therapist (RT), speech-language pathologist (SLP), critical care nurse, and critical care physician. Although each has a well-defined role, there is considerable overlap. Communication and cooperation are essential in providing comprehensive, high-quality care to ICU patients with tracheostomies.

The otolaryngologist is an indispensable member of the team with several responsibilities. These begin at the time of initial consultation with an assessment of the indications and timing of tracheostomy. Preoperative knowledge of the patient's medical history, current illnesses, and medications is essential in optimizing any factors that might otherwise affect the outcome of the procedure adversely. Informed consent must be obtained. The surgeon provides the technical expertise for the operation and decides whether the tracheostomy is best performed percutaneously at the bedside or using a standard open technique in the operating room. A tracheostomy tube with the appropriate characteristics (diameter, length, cuff) is chosen based on the patient's individual needs. Careful follow-up is necessary for the diagnosis and treatment of any immediate or delayed postoperative complications. The otolaryngologist may assess the upper airway prior to decannulation and standardize a decannulation protocol. Finally, the surgeon serves as both an educator and technical resource for the other team members.

The RT is involved in every aspect of tracheostomy care, from the surgical procedure to decannulation. His or her participation in bedside PCT is essential and consists of maintaining adequate ventilation during ET tube manipulation and preventing accidental extubation. Following placement of the tracheostomy tube, the RT continues to adjust ventilator settings in response to the evolving clinical situation. The use of cuffed tubes is frequently necessary, and cuff pressures must be closely monitored so as not to exceed mucosal capillary perfusion pressure. With a tracheostomy in place, the RT may institute and aggressively pursue a protocol to allow weaning in mechanically ventilated patients. The RT participates actively in tracheostomy care and hygiene, including frequency and technique of suctioning and prevention of infection. A great deal of this information is shared and exchanged with the nurse. The RT may also advise on tracheostomy tube type, size, and cuff. In addition the RT can recognize the need for communication and initiate or help institute appropriate plans in this regard. With sufficient clinical improvement, the RT may assist in the decannulation process, assessing the patient's ability to tolerate downsizing and occlusion of the tracheostomy tube.

The SLP promotes the need for effective communication and is therefore often the first to evaluate the patient with a tracheostomy and to suggest the most appropriate form of rehabilitation. In doing so, the SLP assesses the individual's cognitive and linguistic skills and how they can best be used in the context of the clinical setting. Before establishing the best form of communication, the SLP may seek the otolaryngologist's assistance in confirming that the upper airway is patent and physiologically intact. Where clinically possible, cuffed tracheostomy tubes may be exchanged for cuffless tubes, allowing for speech either by manual occlusion of the tube on expiration or by placement of a device such as a Passy-Muir valve. Successful implementation of communication strategies and/or devices depends on detailed instruction, as well as encouragement and support by the SLP toward the nursing staff, patient, and family. The SLP also is involved in monitoring the patient's progress, as well as "troubleshooting" to quickly resolve any difficulties that may arise. The patient

with a tracheostomy frequently has some degree of dysphagia, which is even more pronounced when mechanical ventilation is required. The SLP frequently is called upon for the initial assessment of swallowing dysfunction and may provide expertise for rehabilitation in a number of different areas, including food consistencies, head position, and swallowing sequences.

The critical care nurse is intimately involved in every aspect of tracheostomy care. Following placement of the tracheostomy tube, the nurse may be the first to recognize any procedure-related complications, such as subcutaneous emphysema, excessive ventilatory pressures from pneumothorax, and obstruction of the tracheobronchial tree with blood and secretions. These difficulties are then brought to the attention of the critical care physician and dealt with appropriately.

Consistently high standards of nursing care are key in ensuring good tracheostomy hygiene and preventing complications. Timely changes of soiled tracheostomy ties, frequent cleaning of the surgical site, and attention to the neckplate-skin interface all minimize the likelihood of skin maceration, breakdown, and wound infection. Continuous high humidity, judicious suctioning utilizing proper technique, and frequent cleaning and/or changing of the inner cannula effectively prevents the formation of mucous plugs.

The nurse works closely with the SLP in encouraging communication and also with the RT in implementing good tracheostomy care and facilitating the weaning process. To those patients who are not ventilator-dependent, when their condition permits, the nurse may offer instruction in tracheostomy self-care.

The nurse also participates in the decannulation process by providing ongoing tracheostomy care and ensuring adequate closure of the stoma.

The critical care physician is at the head of the team and is responsible for providing the best possible tracheostomy care by encouraging participation, communication, and cooperation among the various members of the team. In consultation with the surgeon, the physician decides on both the need and timing for a tracheostomy. Decisions regarding tracheostomy tube type, dimensions, and cuff pressures are individualized according to the patient's needs. The critical care physician may see the placement of a tracheostomy as facilitating the pursuit of certain goals in patient care. These may include more rapid weaning or aggressive pulmonary toilet. Success in these areas may, in turn, allow eventual decannulation and closure of the tracheostomy.

The critical care physician is also responsible for the patient's nutritional needs. Dysphagia, a common problem, must be investigated and, when possible, treated. Frequently the necessary calories must be delivered by the enteral or parenteral route, at least temporarily. The critical care physician discusses treatment goals with the team members and oversees and assists their efforts at providing comprehensive care.

REFERENCES

1. Zeitouni A, Kost K. Tracheostomy: a retrospective review of 281 patients. *J Otolaryngol*. 1994;23:61–66.
2. Stauffer JN, Olson DE, Petty TL. Complications and consequences of endotracheal intubation and tracheostomy: prospective study of 150 critically ill adult patients. *Am J Med*. 1981;70:65–76.
3. Indeck M, Peterson S, Smith J, et al. Risk, cost and benefit of transporting ICU patients for special studies. *J Trauma*. 1988;28:1020–1025.
4. Smith I, Fleming S, Cernaianu A. Mishaps during transport from the intensive care unit. *Crit Care Med*. 1990;18:278–281.
5. Waddell G. Movement of critically ill patients within hospital. *Br Med J*. 1975;2:417–419.
6. Taylor JO, Landers CF, Chulay JD, Hood WB, Abelmann WH. Monitoring high-risk cardiac patients during transportation in hospital. *Lancet*. 1997;2(7685):1205–1208.
7. Seldinger SI. Catheter replacement of the needle in percutaneous arteriography. *Acta Radiol*.1953;39:368–376.
8. Shelden CH, Pudenz RH, Fresshwater DB, Crue BL. A new method for tracheostomy. *J Neurosurg*. 1955;12:428–431.
9. Schachner A, Ovil Y, Sidi J, Rogev M, Heilbronn Y, Levy MJ. Percutaneous tracheostomy—a new method. *Crit Care Med*. 1989;17:1052-1056.
10. Toye FJ, Weinstein JD. A percutaneous tracheostomy device. *Surgery*. 1969;65:384–389.
11. Ciaglia P, Firsching R, Syniec C. Elective percutaneous dilatational tracheostomy. A new simple bedside procedure; preliminary report. *Chest*. 1985;87:715–719.
12. Wang MB, Berke GS, Ward PH, Calcaterra TC, Watts D. Early experience with percutaneous tracheostomy. *Laryngoscope*. 1992;102:157-162.
13. Marelli D, Paul A, Manolidis S, et al. Endoscopic guided percutaneous tracheostomy: early results of a consecutive trial. *J Trauma*. 1990;30:433-435.
14. Kost K. Percutaneous tracheostomy. *Laryngoscope* (suppl). 2005;115:1-30.
15. Kost KM. The optimal technique of percutaneous tracheostomy. *Int J Intensive Care*. 2001;8:82-88.

16. Dayal VS, Masri WE. Tracheostomy in intensive care setting. *Laryngoscope.* 1986;96:58–60.

17. Astrachan DI, Kirchner JC, Goodwin WJ. Prolonged intubation versus tracheostomy: complications, practical and psychological considerations. *Laryngoscope.* 1988;98:1165–1169.

18. Hazard P, Jones C, Bernitone J. Comparative clinical trial of standard operative tracheostomy with percutaneous tracheostomy. *Crit Care Med.* 1991;19: 1018–1024.

19. Friedman Y, Fildes J, Mizock B, et al. Comparison of percutaneous and surgical tracheostomies. *Chest.* 1996;110:480–485.

20. Gysin C, Dulguerov P, Guyot J-P, Perneger TV, Abajo B, Chevrolet J-C. Percutaneous versus surgical tracheostomy: a double blind randomized trial. *Ann Surg.* 1999; 230:708–714.

21. Futran ND, Dutcher PO, Roberts JK. The safety and efficacy of bedside tracheostomy. *Otolaryngol Head Neck Surg.* 1993;109:707–711.

22. Wease GL, Frikker M, Villalba M, Glover J. Bedside tracheostomy in the intensive care unit. *Arch Surg.* 1996;131:552–555.

23. Stock MC, Woodward CG, Shapiro BA, Cane RD, Lewis V, Pecaro B. Perioperative complications of elective tracheostomy in critically ill patients. *Crit Care Med.* 1986;14:861–863.

24. Goldstein SI, Breda SD, Schneider KL. Surgical complications of bedside tracheostomy in an otolaryngology residency program. *Laryngoscope.* 1987;97: 1407–1409.

25. Porter JM, Ivatury RR. Preferred route of tracheostomy—percutaneous versus open at the bedside: a randomized, prospective study in the surgical intensive care unit. *Am Surg.* 1999;65: 142–146.

26. Dulguerov P, Gysin C, Perneger TV, Chevrolet JC. Percutaneous or surgical tracheostomy: a meta-analysis. *Crit Care Med.* 1999;27:1617–1625.

27. Winkler WB, Karnik R, Seelmann O, et al. Bedside percutaneous tracheostomy with endoscopic guidance: experience with 71 ICU patients. *Intens Care Med.* 1994;20: 476–479.

28. Barba CA, Angood PB, Kauder DR, et al. Bronchoscopic guidance makes percutaneous tracheostomy a safe cost-effective, and easy-to-teach procedure. *Surgery.* 1995;118:879–883.

29. Polderman KH, Spijkstra JJ, de Bree R, et al. Percutaneous tracheostomy in the intensive care unit: which safety precautions? *Crit Care Med.* 2001;29:221–223.

30. Dexter TJ. A cadaver study appraising accuracy of blind placement of percutaneous tracheostomy. *Anesthesia.* 1995; 50:863–864.

31. Anderson HL, Bartlett RH. Elective tracheostomy for mechanical ventilation by the percutaneous technique. *Clin Chest Med.*;12:555–560.

32. Grantcharov TP, Bardam L, Funch-Jensen P, Rosenberg J. Learning curves and impact of previous operative experience on performance on a virtual reality simulator to test laparoscopic surgical skills. *Am J Surg.* 2003;185:146–149.

33. Stowe DG, Kenen PD, Hudson WR. Complications of tracheostomy. *Am Surg.* 1970;36:34–37.

34. Golz A, Goldsher M, Eliachar I, Joachims HZ. Fatal haemorrhage following a misplaced tracheostomy. *J Laryngol Otol.* 1981;95:529–533.

35. Bernard SA, Jones BM, Shearer WA. Percutaneous dilatational tracheostomy complicated by delayed life-threatening haemorrhage. *Aust N Z J Surg.* 1992; 62:152–153.

36. Shlugman D, Satya-Krishna R, Loh L. Acute fatal haemorrhage during percutaneous dilatational tracheostomy. *Br J Anaesth.* 2003;90:517–520.

37. Goldenberg D, Golz A, Netzer A, Joachims HZ. Tracheostomy: changing indications and a review of 1130 cases. *J Otolaryngol.* 2002;31:211–215.

38. Fradis M, Malatskey S, Dor I, et al. Early complications of tracheostomy performed in the operating room. *J Otolaryngol.* 2003;12:55-57.

39. Marx WH, Ciaglia P, Graniero KD. Some important details in the technique of percutaneous dilatational tracheostomy via the modified Seldinger technique. *Chest.* 1996;110:763-766.

40. Massick DD, Yao S, Powell DM, et al. Bedside tracheostomy in the intensive care unit: a prospective randomized trial comparing open surgical tracheostomy with endoscopically guided percutaneous dilatational tracheostomy. *Laryngoscope.* 2001;111:494-500.

41. Friedman Y, Mayer AD. Bedside percutaneous tracheostomy in critically ill patients. *Chest.* 1993;104:532-535.

42. Fischler MP, Kuhn M, Cantieni R, Frutiger A. Late outcome of percutaneous dilatational tracheostomy in intensive care patients. *Intens Care Med.* 1995;21:475-481.

43. Rosenbower TJ, Morris JA, Eddy VA, Ries WR. The long-term complications of percutaneous dilatational tracheostomy. *Am Surg.* 1998;64:82-87.

44. Upadhyay A, Maurer J, Turner J, Tiszenkel H, Rosengart T. Elective bedside tracheostomy in the intensive care unit. *J Am Coll Surg.* 1996;183:51-55.

45. Toursarkissian B, Zweng T, Kearney P, et al. Percutaneous dilational tracheostomy: report of 141 cases. *Ann Thorac Surg.* 1994;57:862-867.

46. Ciaglia P, Graniero KD. Percutaneous dilatational tracheostomy: Results and long-term follow-up. *Chest.* 1992;101:464-467.

47. Bodenham A, Diament R, Cohen A, Webster N. Percutaneous dilatational tracheostomy: a bedside procedure in the intensive care unit. *Anaesthesia.* 1991; 46:570-572.

48. Blankenship DR, Gourin CG, Davis B, et al. Percutaneous tracheostomy: don't beat them, join them. *Laryngoscope.* 2004;114:1517-1521.

49. Freeman BD, Isabella K, Lin N, Buchman TG. A meta-analysis of prospective trials comparing percutaneous and surgical tracheostomy in critically ill patients. *Chest.* 2000;118:1412-1418.

50. Yaremchuk K. Regular tracheostomy tube changes to prevent formation of granulation tissue. *Laryngoscope.* 2003; 113:1-10.

51. Florete OG, Kirby RR. Airway management. In: Civetta JM, Taylor RW, Kirby RR, eds. *Critical Care.* Philadelphia, Pa: Lippincott-Raven; 1997:757-776.

52. Heffner JE, Miller KS, Sahn SA. Tracheostomy in the intensive care unit: complications. *Chest.* 1986;90:430-436.

53. Bernhard WN, Yost L, Joynes D, et al. Intracuff pressures in endotracheal and tracheostomy tubes. *Chest.* 1985;87: 720-725.

54. Young PJ, Pakeerathan S, Blunt MC, Subramanya S. A low-volume, low-pressure tracheal tube cuff reduces pulmonary aspiration. *Crit Care Med.* 2006;34: 632-639.

55. Clarke L. A critical event in tracheostomy care. *Br J Nurs.* 1995;4:676-681.

56. Hooper M. Nursing care of the patient with a tracheostomy. *Nurs Stand.* 1996; 10:40-43.

57. Fowler S, Knapp-Spooner C, Donnohue D. The ABCs of tracheostomy care. *J Prac Nurs.* 1995;45:44-48.

58. Deppe SA, Kelly JW, Thoi LL, et al. Incidence of colonization, nosocomial pneumonia, and mortality in critically ill patients using a Trach-Care closed-suction system versus an open-suction system: prospective, randomized study. *Crit Care Med.* 1990;18:1389-1393.

59. Karnad DR, Mhaisekar DG, Moralwar KV. Respiratory mucus pH in tracheostomized intensive care patients: effects of colonization and pneumonia. *Crit Care Med.* 1990;18:699-701.

60. McKenney MG, Norwood S. The prevalence and importance of nosocomial infections in the intensive care unit. In:

Civetta JM, Taylor RW, Kirby RR, eds. *Critical Care*. Philadelphia, Pa: Lippincott-Raven; 1997:1573-1588.

61. George DL. Epidemiology of nosocomial pneumonia in intensive care unit patients. *Clin Chest Med*. 1995;16: 26-44.

62. Sottile FD, Marrie TJ, Prough DS et al. Nosocomial pulmonary infection: Possible etiologic significance of bacterial adhesion to endotracheal tubes. *Crit Care Med*. 1986;14:265-270.

63. Snow N, Richardson JD, Flint LM. Management of necrotizing tracheostomy infections. *J Thorac Cardiovasc Surg*. 1981;82:341-44.

64. Potgieter PD, Linton DM, Oliver S, Forder AA. Nosocomial infections in a respiratory intensive care unit. *Crit Care Med*. 1987;15:495-498.

65. Pawar M, Mehta Y, Khurana P, Chaudhary A, Kulkarni V, Trehan N. Ventilator-associated pneumonia: incidence, risk factors, outcome, and microbiology. *J Cardiothorac Vasc Anesth*. 2003;17:22-28.

66. Talep K, Getch CL, Criner GJ. Swallowing dysfunction in patients receiving prolonged mechanical ventilation. *Chest*. 1996;109:167-172.

67. Marian M, Rappaport W, Cunningham D, et al. The failure of conventional methods to promote spontaneous transpyloric feeding tube passage and the safety of intragastric feeding in the critically ill ventilated patient. *Surg Gynecol Obstet*. 1993;176:475-479.

68. Moore FA, Haenel JB, Moore EE, Read RA. Percutaneous tracheostomy/gastrostomy in brain-injured patients—a minimally invasive alternative. *J Trauma*. 1992;33: 435-439.

69. Montecalvo MA, Stegler KA, Farber HW, et al. Nutritional outcome and pneumonia in critical care patients randomized to gastric versus jejunal tube feedings. *Crit Care Med*. 1992;20:1377-1387.

70. Whatley K, Turner WW, Dey M, et al. Transpyloric passage of feeding tubes. *Nutr Supp Serv*. 1983;3:18-21.

CHAPTER 6

Selecting a Tracheostomy Tube: Current Options

CARL-ERIC LINDHOLM

The purpose of a tracheostomy tube is (1) to provide a secure continuation of the airway through the passage of the soft tissues of the neck; (2) to offer a possibility of artificial positive pressure ventilation if needed; and (3) to seal the trachea to prevent aspiration of material above the tube or in the hypopharynx. Because the materials used and design of the tube may differ according to its intended use, it is necessary to determine what mandatory and optional functions the tube should perform before it is inserted. For instance, if the patient can protect his airway against aspiration by sphincter action of the larynx, an uncuffed tube is generally sufficient, whereas if positive pressure ventilation is needed or the patient is unable to protect the airway against aspiration, it is necessary to use a cuffed tube.

Most tracheostomy tubes can be used either for conventional surgical tracheotomy or percutaneous tracheotomy. Special equipment is needed for the percutaneous tracheotomy and is available from major tube manufacturers, who deliver kits for the procedure.

TUBE MATERIALS

Silver has long been used to manufacture tracheostomy tubes because the metal walls of the tube can be kept very thin, which is especially advantageous when an inner cannula is used (Fig 6-1). In addition silver has antibacterial properties. However, the rigidity of metal tubes and their shape created problems. For this reason, rubber began to be used to make tracheostomy tubes, and by 1871 Trendelburg[1] had constructed a tube with a cuff of this material. Latex, as well as red rubber, has largely given way to polyvinyl chloride (PVC) and similar materials today because plastics can be manufactured to obtain tubes of varying degrees of rigidity. For instance, a tube of

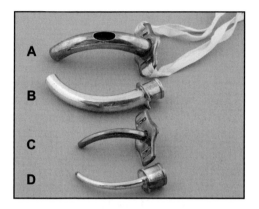

Fig 6–1. The old silver tracheostomy tubes. **A.** Fenestrated tube. **B.** Inner tube with nonstandard connector. **C.** Small size pediatric tube. **D.** Inner tube not fenestrated with nonstandard connector.

pronounced flexibility which does not collapse can be produced if the wall of the tube is reinforced by a spiral of more rigid material (Fig 6-2). Such a tube is especially useful when airway anatomy is abnormal as the tube can adapt to the configuration of the airway.[2] Cuffed tubes can be made by bonding a cuff of strong but extremely thin material to a tube made of similar material. Because silicone is inert, it is a desirable material for tracheostomy tubes, but it is difficult to produce a large resting-diameter silicone cuff with a thin wall which is of acceptably low distensibility. In addition, it is very difficult to attach other cuff materials securely to a silicone tube. For this reason, tracheostomy tubes continue to be made of a variety of materials.

Nevertheless, the material chosen must meet certain specifications. The tube and cuff surface should be smooth, and all tube and cuff materials should be biocompatible and pass the implantation test described in the U.S. Pharmacopeia or other relevant national regulation,

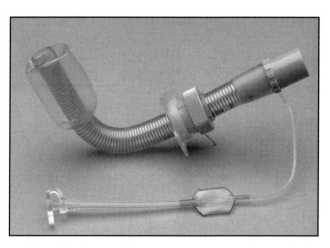

Fig 6–2. Reinforced flexible tracheostomy tube (Rusch) with movable neck plate, which can be locked at suitable level. The drawback with this design is that the machine end of the tube often is protruding too far from the neck.

depending on the country. Finally, the tube should be radiopaque or have a radiopaque indicator which will be visible on a radiograph.

TUBE DESIGN

Connector

Tracheostomy tubes for adults should have a male 15-mm conical connector (ISO 5366-1:2000).[3] The connector is mostly bonded to the outer tube (Fig 6–3). Some tubes, however, have the connector bonded to the inner tube, which thus has to be in situ during ventilator treatment (Fig 6–4).

Shape

There are two main designs of tracheostomy tubes, those which are shaped like a quarter arc of a circle (curved tubes; see Fig 6–3), and those which are angled to fit the trachea at one end and the area between the skin and the trachea at the other (see Fig 6–4). The midportions of angled tubes are smoothly curved and have rather small diameters. The angle between the limbs is usually obtuse and may be stated by the manufacturer, which is of help in choosing the proper tube for each patient.

The quarter-circle tracheostomy tubes usually have an inner portion which can be removed and cleaned while the outer

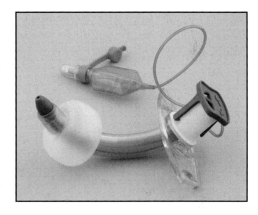

Fig 6–3. Curved tracheostomy tube (Portex) with introducer (obturator) in situ and with 15-mm connector.

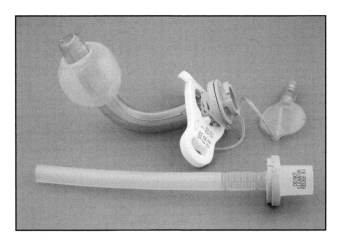

Fig 6–4. Angled tracheostomy tube (Shiley) with straight flexible inner tube with bonded 15-mm connector. When in situ the inner tube is locked to the outer tube.

tube remains in situ. This is an advantage when inexperienced personnel must take care of the tracheostomy or when the patient must do it him- or herself, for example, in chronic cases. In addition, the outer tube may be fenestrated to permit speech when the inner portion is removed, although when the inner tube is inserted, the entire system functions as an unfenestrated tube (provided there are no granulations in the window and the outer tube is reasonably clean) (Fig 6-5). Some tubes are also delivered with an inner part which also has a window corresponding to that of the outer tube (see Fig 6-5). Unfortunately, the window in fenestrated tubes is often placed too near the neck plate; it may be desirable in some cases to obtain a plastic two-piece tube of this design without a window and then to cut a window at the desired location.

Nevertheless, curved tubes have many disadvantages. Because the curved tube enters the tracheal wall at a more acute angle than an angled tube the hole in the trachea will be oval, with its longest dimension along the longitudinal axis of the trachea; thus, insertion of such a tube may require transection of another tracheal cartilage. In addition, curved tubes tend to compress the anterior tracheal wall immediately above the stoma, which in time leads to indentation of the tracheal wall and sometimes to destruction of the anterior part of the cartilage next to the upper border of the tracheostomy. This results in further longitudinal extension of the defect in the tracheal wall. Another disadvantage of curved tubes is that because the intratracheal part of the tube is an arc of a circle and the trachea is mostly straight, the tube often does not conform to the trachea. The convex part of the tube may compress the membranous part of the trachea, with risk of a tracheoesophageal fistula, whereas the tube tip may traumatize the anterior tracheal wall with lethal penetration to the innominate artery (Fig 6-6).

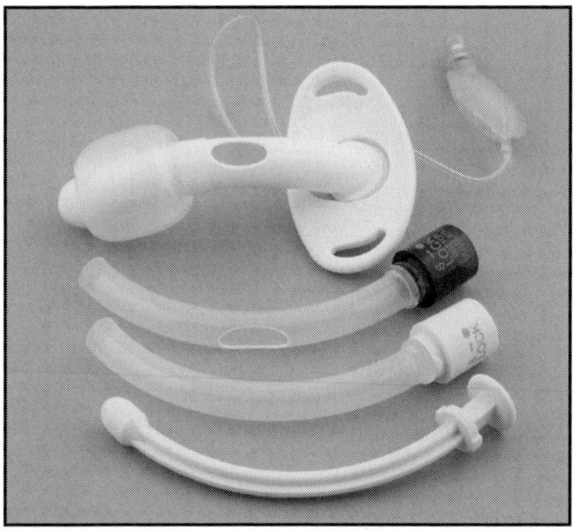

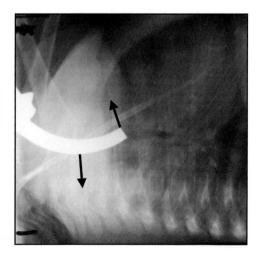

Fig 6–6. Lateral radiograph of a child's neck and chest showing the position of the curved tube. Note that the edge of the tube tip is pressing on the anterior tracheal wall and that the convexity seems to compress the posterior membraneous part of the trachea (*arrows show direction of pressure*).

Fig 6–5. Fenestrated curved tracheostomy tube (Shiley) with fenestrated and unfenestrated inner tubes with 15-mm connector and introducer (obturator).

Angled tracheostomy tubes have many advantages over those just described. The transmural limb enters the trachea at a less acute angle than it does in curved tubes, so that the hole in the trachea is almost round, and usually only two tracheal cartilages rather than three will lose their anterior part and their arch function. In addition, angled tubes exert less pressure on the anterior tracheal wall above the stoma, and because the straight intratracheal limb is usually well centered in the trachea, the threat of pressure necrosis of the tracheal wall is much less with the angled tube than with the curved tubes (see also under "New Development").

One disadvantage of using angled tubes is that it is difficult to fit such tubes with inner tubes, which must be flexible to slip into position. Such tubes are available, however (see Fig 6-4). When tubes with inner portions are used, it must be kept in mind that they will take up more space in the air passage: although tube size is generally designated by the inside diameter (ID) of the outer tube, the manufacturer must also give the inside diameter of the inner tube, which is to be considered when choosing the tube.

Neck Plate

The neck plate of the tracheostomy tube should be securely attached to the tube so that it can keep the tube in position. The neck plate is usually straight and attaches at a 90° angle to the tube (see Fig 6-2), which usually fits the average person well. However, for a patient with a short neck or an infant it is less satisfactory, and in such patients tubes with an Aberdeen[4] neck plate, which looks like an airplane wing, is much more comfortable to the neck (see Pediatric Trache-

ostomy Tubes). This neck plate has for a long time been used on some pediatric plastic, as well as silicone, tracheostomy tubes, and a similar design also is now used on some tracheostomy tubes for adults. Although the distance from the skin to the trachea (transmural distance) differs in the population, the standard distance from the neck plate to the intratracheal limb usually fits patients whose anatomy is normal.

However, if the transmural distance in the patient is shorter than normal and the straps around the neck force the neck plate against the skin, the intratracheal part of the tube does not conform properly to the trachea, and tracheal lesions of the same kind as seen with curved tubes may occur. Conversely, if the patient's transmural distance is greater than average, the tube will exert pressure against the inside of the anterior wall of the trachea near the lower border of the tracheostomy and cause damage. Some tubes have adjustable neck plates, which partly solves this problem (see Fig 6-2).

An adjustable neck plate is slid up or down the transmural part of the tracheostomy tube to the desired position and then secured by a neck plate lock (see Fig 6-2). A disadvantage by this design is that the long machine end of the tube is sticking out too far from the neck, the effect of which is that the tube may be tilted by a ventilator tubing with a potential risk of tracheal damage. Another concept is to make tubes with different transmural lengths of the same tube size (see New Development).

Uncuffed Tubes

The uncuffed tubes are made of the same material and have the same size range and shapes as cuffed tubes (Fig 6-7).

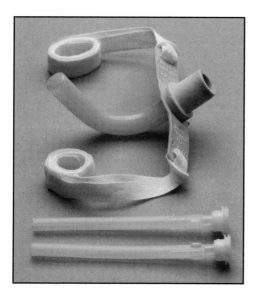

Fig 6–7. Example of an uncuffed tracheostomy tube (Portex) of the angled type with neck straps tied to the neck plate and two flexible inner tubes.

They are mostly used when the patient has spontaneous respiration and is able to protect his or her airway. It is an advantage if an inner tube can be used to facilitate cleaning, especially if the patient him- or herself is supposed to do so.

Cuffs

Slip-on cuffs should not be used as they may slip off the tracheostomy tube during use and occlude the trachea distal to the tube. A large variety of cuffs are available. Air- or gas-filled cuffs are most commonly used and it is generally agreed that small resting-diameter, small residual-volume, high-pressure cuffs should be abandoned[5-15] in favor of large resting-diameter, large residual-volume, low-pressure cuffs, with a thin wall.

To function as a large resting-diameter cuff, the cuff should have a circumference at rest well exceeding that of the trachea in which it is placed at the recommended intracuff pressure. That is, when the cuff is inflated to the recommended pressure, it should drape even irregular tracheas and be slightly folded within the trachea. For instance, the resting diameter of cuffs used on tubes for adults should have a resting diameter of approximately 30 mm[5,11,15,16] (that is, when inflated to a pressure of 20 mm H_2O) to meet the above criteria with some safety margin.

Cuffs with thinner walls have been preferred because large resting-diameter cuffs with thick walls have been shown to have elevated pressures at the ridges of the folds and also to create channels through which liquid from above the cuff may flow to contaminate the lower airways. These thin-walled cuffs conform better to the tracheal wall and provide a better seal, thus affording better protection from aspiration.[17] An ultrathin cuff drapes the irregularities of the tracheal mucosa and exerts a more evenly distributed pressure, which saves the microcirculation and minimizes development of lesions of the tracheal wall.[13,18]

The maximum length of the cuff is limited by the length of the intratracheal portion of the tracheostomy tube, whereas the minimum cuff length which is functional depends upon the outer diameter of the cuff. Generally, the cuff on tubes for adults is between 20 and 30 mm long, whereas cuffs are proportionally shorter for smaller tubes; so far there is no evidence that the shape of the cuff alone (cylindrical, rounded, or pear-shaped) has any bearing on its performance or potential to traumatize the trachea.

A different type of cuff has been developed which has special features. A large resting-diameter silicone cuff filled with plastic foam was designed by

Kamen and Wilkinson[19] (Fig 6–8). Before insertion of this tracheostomy tube, air in the cuff must be evacuated with a syringe connected to the cuff-deflating tube. This causes atmospheric pressure to compress the foam so that the tube may be inserted through the tracheostomy. When the cuff is in the trachea, the cuff-deflating tube is left open and when air pressure equilibrates, the compressed foam will expand owing to its elasticity and create a seal in the trachea.

Cuff-Inflating Tube and Pilot Balloon

The tube through which the cuff is inflated is generally connected to a sep- arate lumen within the tube wall near the machine end of the tracheostomy tube, whereas the other end of the lumen is open inside the cuff. It is advantageous if the inflation tube has more than one opening within the cuff, so that if one of the openings should be occluded by the thin cuff wall during evacuation of cuff air, the cuff could still be deflated. The free end of the inflating tubes should have a connector which fits a conical male Luer connector. It can be sealed with a simple plug (see Fig 6–2) or, as in most modern tracheostomy tubes, with a closure valve which is an integral part of the Luer connector (see Fig 6–3). In addition, the inflating tube should contain a balloon to indicate roughly how much the cuff is inflated

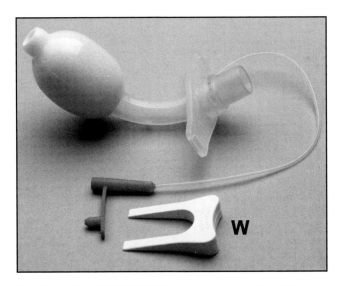

Fig 6–8. The FOAM-CUFF tracheostomy tube (Bivona). The plastic foam in the cuff is self-expanding. Before insertion of the tube, the air in the cuff must be evacuated with a syringe. The cuff is then compressed by atmospheric pressure. When in situ in the trachea, the block (syringe) is removed from the cuff-deflating tube and the cuff expands owing to the elastic recoil of the plastic foam and provides a seal. The wedge (*W*), for easy disconnection of the male and female 15-mm connectors, comes with each tracheostomy tube.

(see Fig 6–2). This so-called pilot balloon also can be a direct continuation of the closure valve (see Fig 6–3).

Cuff Pressure Regulation

A small-resting-diameter cuff must be distended to seal the trachea, but the pressure necessary to overcome the elasticity of the cuff wall varies in different makes. In addition, because the trachea is not circular, pressure of the cuff on the wall varies from area to area,[15,16] so that before a seal is created the trachea must be deformed more or less to the shape of the rather hard cuff and not vice versa.

The pressure exerted against the tracheal wall by a thin-walled, large resting-diameter cuff, on the other hand, is equal to the intracuff pressure and is thus both easy to measure with a simple manometer connected to the cuff-inflating tube via a three-way stopcock and easy to adjust by injecting or removing air with a syringe.[20] Pressure should be checked when the cuff is inflated and at regular intervals and should be kept between 20 and 30 cm H_2O to create a reliable seal for both ventilation and protection from aspiration.[14]

There have been several attempts to develop automatic cuff pressure regulators.[21] McGinnis et al constructed a "pressure-limiting balloon" to be incorporated into the cuff-inflating tube system to keep cuff pressure between 20 and 30 cm H_2O.[22,23] The balloon is made of thin latex and starts to expand when the pressure in the cuff (and cuff-inflating tube) exceeds 20 to 30 cm H_2O, thus preventing further pressure increase in the cuff. To prevent ventilator peak inflation pressure exceeding 20 to 30 cm H_2O to squeeze cuff gas back into the latex balloon, a partial back valve is placed between the latex balloon and the cuff. The latex balloon is protected by a larger, thick-walled open plastic balloon (Fig 6–9). If the latex balloon is inflated to the point at which it reaches the outer plastic balloon the pressure-limiting function will cease. In addition, accidental compression of the balloon, for instance by the head or shoulder of an unconscious patient, must also be avoided, as under certain circumstances the gas in the balloon could be forced into the cuff, causing elevated cuff-to-tracheal wall pressure.

The function of the large resting-diameter silicone cuff filled with plastic foam (see Fig 6–8) has already been mentioned.[19] Because its expansion is self-limiting, it does not cause tracheal dilatation, which may be of special advantage if the trachea has suffered primary damage, for example, due to burn injuries. Its self-limiting expansion is thus a safety factor. However, after some time at body temperature the foam filling the cuff may decrease its elasticity and the seal will loosen. If the cuff is used in a burned trachea, this air leak must be accepted as long as sufficient ventilation can be maintained, whereas such an air leak is actually desirable if the patient shows evidence of tracheal dilatation and signs of imminent tracheal rupture. The cuff deflation tube should never be used to inflate the cuff and should always be left open during use.

Because human tracheas differ in diameter,[16] it is harder to choose the optimal size foam cuff than to choose a suitable large resting-diameter cuff intended to be filled with gas to a desired pressure. Neverthelesss, the manufacturer of the foam cuff (Bivona Surgical Instruments, Hammond, Ind) provides guidelines for choosing tube-cuff sizes for tracheas of different diameters. A simple x-ray mea-

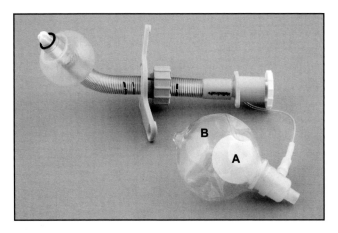

Fig 6–9. The McGinnis pressure-limiting balloon (*A*) (Mallinckrodt) is incorporated in the cuff-inflating tube. When inflation pressure exceeds a value of between 20 and 30 cm H_2O the latex balloon expands and prevents the cuff pressure from increasing further. A special valve keeps the cuff from deflating during short periods of intratracheal peak pressure exceeding 20 to 30 cm H_2O. The latex balloon is enclosed in an open PVC balloon (*B*) for protection; however, the latex balloon will not limit pressure if it is inflated so as to completely fill the PVC balloon. Be sure that the latex balloon is not compressed by pressure from outside as this may result in overinflation of the cuff.

surement of the inner diameter of the trachea may be of help in choosing the appropriate size tube in special patients.

PEDIATRIC TRACHEOSTOMY TUBES

Tracheostomy tubes of less than 5 mm ID are usually supplied without a cuff, and leaks are permitted during ventilation through these tubes, although an unfortunate tendency is to use a tube that fits rather snugly to decrease the leak. A snug-fitting tube has to be chosen when a thick-walled tube is used so that the inner diameter will be sufficient for ventilation. As in either case, however, a large hole in the tracheal wall will result, the chance of post-tracheostomy stomal stenosis is increased. It is still more important to use thin-walled tubes in children than in adults.

Most pediatric tracheostomy tubes are just miniature forms of uncuffed tubes for adults. Physicians are not always as critical as they ought to be when choosing the best tube and demanding more sophisticated pediatric tubes from the manufacturers.

Curved silver tubes have extremely thin walls, and may be used in children, especially if it is felt that an inner tube is necessary. However, the rigid style of these tubes may lead to fatal innominate artery hemorrhage due to tube tip lesions and tracheoesophageal fistula caused by compression of the posterior tracheal wall by the tube (see Fig 6–6). Plastic tubes of the same shape are intended for single use, have thicker walls, and can cause just as much tracheal wall necrosis as silver tubes. Thus, either style is equally undesirable.

Angled pediatric tracheostomy tubes also have essentially the same design as angled adult tubes. Because the distance from the skin to the trachea differs in children, just as it does in adults, the transmural limb may be too short or too long. Thus, it is important not to tie the neck straps too tightly in children fitted with tubes where the transmural limb is a little too long; rather, an extra dressing should be interposed between the skin and the neck plate of the tracheostomy tube, if needed. Children's angled tubes are usually made of plastic or silicone, as are adult tubes, and some made of silicone have the disadvantage discussed above of rather thick walls (Fig 6–10).

In children, and especially in infants, the shape of the neck plate is important. The usual straight neck plates do not fit very well when the neck strap is tied around the neck and tend to pull the tracheostomy tube upward and to tilt the

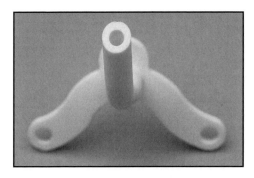

Fig 6–10. Pediatric tracheostomy tube made of silicone with neck plate of Aberdeen design. Example of a tube wall that is too thick.

tube tip anteriorly. The Aberdeen[4] neck plate (see Fig 6–10) conforms much better to the infant neck, and there are tubes on the market made of PVC as well as of silicone with this type of neck plate.

Most pediatric tracheostomy tubes made of plastic or silicone have a 15-mm male standard connector[3] but there are also pediatric tubes with 8-mm connectors and with nonstandard connectors on silver tubes. *The compatibility of the connector on the tracheostomy tube and the ventilator tubing must be ensured before the tracheotomy is started.*

SPECIAL TRACHEOSTOMY TUBES

Some tracheostomy tubes have an extra suction channel incorporated in the tube wall. The suction channel has an opening just above the cuff and continues as a separate suction tube near the machine end of the tracheostomy tube. Aspiration of retained secretions from the trachea above the cuff and in the subglottic area is facilitated. By this arrangement pooling infected secretions may be removed, which decreases the chance of respiratory infection in patients with tracheostomies.[24]

The Kistner tracheostomy tube[25] is a straight conduit made from a serrated cylinder which goes from the skin to just inside the tracheal wall. It comes in four different lengths, with an external diameter of 13.5 mm for adults. In addition a plastic ring can be adjusted around the tube to obtain the needed length for securing it around the neck. Two sizes are available for children. Originally, the Kistner tube was designed to keep a tracheostomy open to facilitate evacuation of retained tracheobronchial secretions.

Presently, it is mostly used to keep a surgically created tracheostomy open for some time following removal of a standard tracheostomy tube, especially when there is doubt that reinsertion of this tube may be necessary.

Other devices with similar functions are the Olympic Trach-Button and a "permanent tracheostomy tube" described by Saul and Bergstrom.[26] The silicone T-tube,[27] all three limbs of which may be cut to desired lengths can, in addition to its use for treatment of tracheal stenosis, be used to secure an alternative airway should the natural airway above the stoma be suspected of providing insufficient air.

For laryngectomy patients there are short silicone tubes with a funnel-shaped outer end instead of a 15-mm connector. The drawbacks with these tubes are that an HMI cannot be connected to them without a 15-mm male connector fitted to the tube.

Phonation

All the above appliances can be equipped with a one-way speech valve, which allows air to enter during inhalation and to be directed through the glottis during exhalation provided the cuff is deflated, and the tube is fenestrated or uncuffed. The one-way valves for these special tubes are usually supplied by the manufacturer of the different tubes. T-tubes must be fitted with a 15-mm male adapter (commonly supplied with endotracheal tubes of different dimensions) before a one-way valve with a standard 15-mm female adapter can be attached.

The so-called Pitt Speaking Tracheostomy Tube[28] (Fig 6–11) is equipped with a separate narrow tube, half of which is incorporated as an additional channel in the tube wall and which ends on the outside of the tube just above the cuff. Oxygen or air at 4 to 6 L/min is delivered through

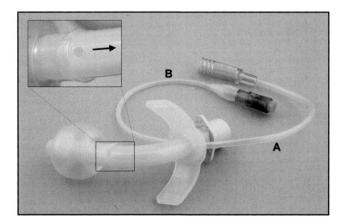

Fig 6–11. The "Pitt Speaking Tracheostomy Tube" (Mallinckrodt). This tube is equipped with a separate tube (*A*) connected to a lumen within the tube wall. This lumen ends on the outside of the tube wall just above the cuff. A flow of 4 to 6 L/min of air or oxygen can be delivered through this line and is forced up through the glottis (*arrow*), making phonation possible even under intermittent positive pressure ventilation. The cuff-inflating tube is also shown (*B*).

this separate tube and is forced up through the glottis as the cuff seals the trachea, thus permitting phonation. In conscious patients treated by ongoing mechanical ventilation, this need for verbal communication should be borne in mind.

This tube design, slightly altered, has also become popular for aspiration of secretion above the cuff (see under Special Tracheostomy Tubes).

OTHER CONSIDERATIONS

Size

The nominal inside diameter (ID) in millimeters of tracheostomy tubes made of plastic is their designated size. Each manufacturer should mark the size of the tube (ID) and also the outside diameter (OD) in millimeters as a guide to the user. In addition, the French gauge (FG or FR), which is three times the outside diameter in millimeters, is often given. The approximate outer diameters and corresponding French gauges for tubes of different inner diameters are given in Table 6–1. If an inner tube is used, the package in which the latter comes should have the size and make of the tube into which it is intended to fit and the inside diameter of the inner tube itself clearly marked. For some reason, manufacturers of metal tubes identify the size of the tube according to the

Table 6–1. Approximate Sizes of Tracheostomy Tubes Made of Plastic

Designated Size = Nominal Inside Diameter	Corresponding Outside Diameter (mm)	French Gauge (FG or FR)
2.5	3.5	FG 11
3.0	4.2	FG 13
3.5	5.0	FG 15
4.0	5.5	FG 17
4.5	6.2	FG 18
5.0	6.7	FG 20
5.5		
6.0	8.0	FG 24
6.5		
7.0	9.3	FG 28
7.5		
8.0	10.7	FG 32
8.5		
9.0	12.0	FG 36
9.5		
10.0	14.0	FG 42

Jackson system, which uses the outer diameter (Table 6–2).

The nominal length of a tracheostomy tube made of plastic is the distance along the center line from the neck plate to the tip. If the neck plate is adjustable, the length varies within a certain range, which may be given by the manufacturer. The nominal length according to the Jackson system is the distance along the inner curvature from the neck plate to the tip.

Sterilization

Disposable tracheostomy tubes are delivered sterile in individual packs marked with the words "sterile" and "for single use." It is important to observe if the pack is intact before it is opened.

Unless the tracheostomy tube is meant for single use, it should be possible to clean, disinfect, and sterilize according to methods recommended by the manufacturer.

Standardization

Currently the International Organization for Standardization (ISO) has issued a standard for connectors on tracheostomy tubes.[3]

Table 6–2. Sizes of Tracheostomy Tubes Made of Metal (Silver)

Designated According to Jackson*	Outside Diameter (mm)	Corresponding French Gauge (FG or FR)
00	4.3	FG 13
0	5.0	FG 15
1	5.5	FG 16.5
2	6.0	FG 18
3	7.0	FG 21
4	8.0	FG 24
5	9.0	FG 27
6	10.0	FG 30
7	11.0	FG 33
8	12.0	FG 36
9	13.0	FG 39
10	14.0	FG 42
11	15.0	FG 45
12	16.0	FG 48

The table is based on information from Pilling Co., Delaware Drive, Fort Washington, Pa 19034.

*The Jackson sizes do not give the inside diameter.

NEW DEVELOPMENT

The Oval Tube

It is clinical knowledge that the destruction of the anterior part of several tracheal cartilages by a tracheostomy sometimes leads to partial collapse and scarring of the trachea during the subsequent heal-ing process following decannulation.[29,30] If, on the contrary, only part of one tracheal cartilage arch has to be resected to accommodate a tube the adjacent intact cartilages will support the scar when healing takes place. Thus, it is less likely that a tracheal stenosis will develop (Fig 6–12).

Based on this observation a new tracheostomy tube (OctaTrach Oval)[31] has been designed to decrease the longi-

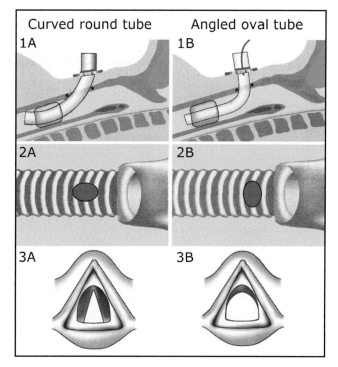

Fig 6–12. 1A. Conventional curved tube in situ. **2A.** Longitudinal defect in the trachea caused by a curved tube. **3A.** If several tracheal cartilage arches have lost their suspending function there is a risk of tracheal collapse. The intact cartilages on both sides of the stoma are located so far apart from each other so they cannot support the part in between: **1B.** Angled tube with oval cross-section in situ. **2B.** The defect in the trachea comprises only part of one tracheal cartilage. **3B.** The two adjacent tracheal cartilages on each side of a short tracheostoma are close to each other and can support the scar tissue during healing and prevent collapse contrary to what can happen when the stoma involves, for example, three cartilages.

tudinal extension of the tracheostoma (Fig 6–13). For the same reason the transmural part of the tube enters the trachea at almost right angles. This tube is now available from the manufacturer (http://www.medprod-octagon.com).

"The Bulged Cuff"

The problem with aspiration of accumulated secretions above the cuff to the lower airways is still a problem in spite of thin large cuffs and a cuff to tracheal pressure of between 20 and 30 cm H_2O. Much effort has been expended to overcome this problem.

Lately, Niels Lomholt in Denmark has developed a thin-walled large-diameter cuff, part of which has several still thinner bubbles in many rows around its circumference (Fig 6–14). In preliminary

tests this design is shown to constitute a better seal in the trachea. This cuff has not yet been marketed but will probably be available soon (Mallinckrodt) if further tests are positive.

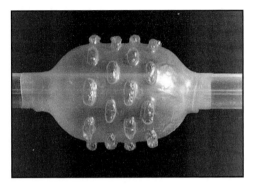

Fig 6–14. The "Bulged Cuff" has a better sealing ability than other cuffs when tested in vitro. It is not yet on the market (Mallinckrodt).

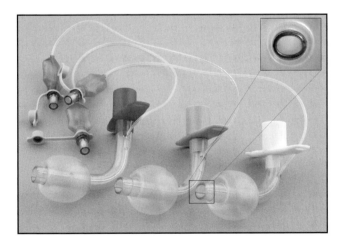

Fig 6–13. The OctaTrach Oval Tracheostomy Tube is designed with an oval cross-section (insert) to save supporting tracheal cartilages. The transmural limb of the tubes differ (Black = long, Gray = medium, White = short) to fit different neck sizes. Medium size tubes usually fit a normal neck. The short tube is suitable for cricothyroidostomy. This tube is new on the market (Medical Products Octagon AB, www.medprod-octagon.com).

CHOOSING THE CORRECT TUBE

General Considerations

The choice of tracheostomy tube is dependent upon many factors. First, the uses to which the tube will be put should be considered, but usually many makes of tubes will meet these criteria. The next consideration is to choose the tubes which cause the least trauma. However, it is necessary to have some selection of tubes in stock in the hospital to meet all the special situations that may arise. If the primary role of the physician, not to harm the patient (*primum est non nocere*), is kept in mind, it should be possible to stock a variety of tubes for different uses but of such type as will cause least trauma to the trachea.

Specific features that are important in preventing harm include the qualities of the cuff and whether or not the tube conforms to the airway anatomy. In addition, consideration should be given as to whether a tube with an inner portion which can be removed easily for cleaning would be desirable; removable inner tubes are useful if the patient uses the tracheostomy tube for a long time at home and must clean tenacious secretions and dry crusts from the tube by him- or herself. On the other hand, if the tracheostomy tube is fitted with a heat-and-moisture exchanger ("artificial nose"), secretions are kept more liquid and are easier to cough up or to remove by suction,[32,33] which makes inner tubes much less important. Finally, inner tubes should not be used in plastic pediatric tracheostomy tubes because they compromise the airway too much. In addition, the thickness of the wall of a silicone tube and the plastic tube should be checked.

Pediatric tracheostomy tubes with neck plates of the Aberdeen design (see Fig 6–10) usually adapt to the neck better than straight neck plates.

Specific Checklist

1. Check type of connector: the fitting on the ventilation system must be one intended to be connected to a tracheostomy tube. A 15-mm male conical fitting is standard on tracheostomy tubes but some pediatric tubes and silver tubes have other fittings.

2. The tracheostomy tube used should not be wider than necessary: for adult males an 8-mm-ID tube (FG 32) and for adult females a 7-mm-ID tube (FG 30) are recommended.

3. The shape of the tracheostomy tube should conform as closely as possible to the anatomy of the airway.

4. Make sure that the cuff, if provided, is securely bonded to the tube and that the cuff and cuff-inflating system are airtight before the tube is inserted into the patient.

5. It is generally agreed that large resting-diameter cuffs should be used. Cuff pressure as measured via the cuff inflating tube is approximately equal to the cuff pressure on the tracheal wall. To reliably function as a large resting-diameter cuff intended for adults the cuff resting diameter should be about 30 mm.

6. The thinner the cuff wall, the lower the effective cuff-to-tracheal wall sealing pressure and thus the less the tracheal wall damage will be and the less the microcircula-

tion of the tracheal mucosa will be compromised.

7. Cuff pressure can be measured with a manometer connected to the cuff-inflating tube via a three-way stopcock. This should be done when the cuff is inflated and whenever indicated thereafter. The cuff-inflating tube can also be continuously connected to a manometer. Adequate intracuff pressure is between 20 and 30 cm H$_2$O. The cuff pressure can also be kept at a desired level by automatic pressure-regulating devices. (the "just seal" or "minimum leak" method is *not* recommended).

REFERENCES

1. Trendelenburg F. Beiträge zu den Operationen an den Luftwegen. *Archiv Klin Chir.* 1871;12:112.
2. Lomholt N, Borgeskov S, Kirby B. A new tracheostomy tube. III. Bronchofiberoptic examination of the trachea after prolonged intubation with the NL tracheostomy tube. *Acta Anaesthesiol Scand.* 1981;25:407-411.
3. International Standards Organization. ISO 2000:5366-1. *Anaesthetic and respiratory equipment—Tracheostomy tubes—Part 1: tubes and connectors for use in adults.* New York, NY: Author.
4. Aberdeen E. Tracheostomy and tracheostomy care in infants. *Proc R Soc Med.* 1965;59:900-902.
5. Lomholt N. A new tracheostomy tube. I. Cuff with controlled pressure on the tracheal mucous membrane. *Acta Anaestheiol Scand* (suppl). 1967;11:311.
6. Geffin B, Pontoppidan H. Reduction of tracheal damage by the prestretching of inflatable cuffs. *Anesthesiology.* 1969; 31:462-463.
7. Carroll RG, Hedden M, Safar P. Intratracheal cuffs: performance characteristics. *Anesthesiology.* 1969; 31:275-281.
8. Cooper JD, Grillo HC. Experimental production and prevention of injury due to cuffed tracheal tubes. *Surg Gynecol Obstet.* 1969;129:1235-1241.
9. Carroll RG. Evaluation of tracheal tube cuff designs. *Crit Care Med* 1973;1:45-46.
10. Grillo HC, Cooper JD, Geffin B, et al. A low-pressure cuff for tracheostomy tubes to minimize tracheal injury. A comparative clinical trial. *J Thorac Cardiovasc Surg.* 1971; 62:898-907.
11. Carroll RG, McGinnis GE, Grenvik A. Performance characteristics of tracheal cuffs. *Int Anesthesiol Clin.* 1974;12:1111-1141.
12. Dane TEB, King EG. A prospective study of complications after tracheostomy for assisted ventilation. *Chest* 1975;67:398-404.
13. Nordin U, Lindholm CE, Wolgast M. Blood flow in the rabbit tracheal mucosa under normal conditions and under the influence of tracheal intubation. *Acta Anaesthesiol Scand.* 1977; 21:81-94.
14. Fruhwald H, Schmiedl R. Cuffschädigungen der Trachealschleimhaut bei Intubation. *Ann Otol Rhinol Laryngol (Stuttg).* 1980;59:737-742.
15. Toty L, Butez J. Le conflict canule-trachée chez les tracheotomisés. *Rev Fr Mal Respir.* 1974;2:361.
16. Mackenzie CF, Shin B, Whitley N, et al. The relationship of human tracheal size to body habitus. *Anesthesiology.* 1979; 51(suppl):378.
17. Bernhard WN, Cottrell JE, Sivakumaran C, et al: Adjustment of intracuff pressure to prevent aspiration. *Anesthesiology.* 1979;50:363-366.
18. Nordin U, Engstrom B, Lindholm CE. Surface structure of the tracheal wall after different duration of intubation. *Acta Otolaryngol Suppl.* 1977;345:59.
19. Kamen JM, Wilkinson CJ. A new low-pressure cuff for endotracheal tubes. *Anesthesiology.* 1971; 34:482-485.

20. Carroll RG, Grenvik A. Proper use of large-diameter large-residual-volume cuffs. *Crit Care Med.* 1973;1:153–154.

21. Lomholt N. A new tracheostomy tube. II. Cuff with self-adjusting minimum pressure on the tracheal mucosa during inspiration and expiration. *Acta Anaesthesiol Scand.* 1971(suppl 44).

22. McGinnis GE, Shively JG, Patterson RL, et al. An engineering analysis of intratracheal tube cuffs. *Anesth Analg (Cleve).* 1971;50:557–564.

23. Magovern GJ, Shively JG, Fecht D, et al. The clinical and experimental evaluation of a controlled-pressure intratracheal cuff. *J Thorac Cardiovasc Surg.* 1972; 64:747–756.

24. Dezfulian C, Shojania K, Collard HR, et al. Subglottic secretion drainage for preventing ventilator-associated pneumonia: a meta-analysis. *Am J Med.* 2005;118:11–18.

25. Kistner RL, Hanlon CR. A new tracheostomy tube in treatment of retained bronchial secretions. *Arch Surg.* 1960; 81:259–262.

26. Saul A, Bergstrom B. A new permanent tracheostomy tube speech valve system. *Laryngoscope.* 1979;89:980–983.

27. Montgomery WW. T-tube tracheal stent. *Arch Otolaryngol.* 1965 82:320–321.

28. Safar P, Grenvik A Speaking cuff tracheostomy tube. *Crit Care Med.* 1975; 3:23–26.

29. Pearsson FG, Goldberg M, da Silva AJ. Tracheal stenosis complicating tracheostomy with cuffed tubes. *Arch Surg.* 1968; 97:380–394.

30. Arola MK, Puhakka H, Mäkelä P. Healing of lesions caused by cuffed tracheostomy tubes and their late sequelae. A follow-up study. *Acta Anaesth Scand.* 1980;24:169–177.

31. Lindholm CE, Randestad A, Gertzen H. New design of a tracheostomy-cricothyroidostomy tube. *Eur Arch Otorhinolaryngol.* 2003;260:421–424.

32. Revenas B, Lindholm CE. The Foam Nose—a new disposable heat and moisture exhanger. A comparison with other similar devices. *Acta Anaesthesiol Scan.* 1979;23:34–39.

33. Revenas B, Lindholm CE. Temperature variations in disposable heat and moisture exchangers. *Acta Anaesthesiol Scand.* 1980;24:237–240.

CHAPTER 7

Tracheostomy in Burn Patients

HARVEY SLATER

Patients suffering thermal burns may also be exposed to superheated gases containing toxic chemical compounds. This may occur in a flash fire that causes burns to the patient's face. This may also occur with entrapment where the patient is unable to avoid flame injury to the face and is forced to take breaths of hot gases prior to rescue or escape. Thermal and chemical injury to the oropharynx causes a rapid change in capillary hemodynamics and transmembrane flux, which results in edema.[1] This edema may rapidly accumulate and cause respiratory obstruction. The severity of the edema and the rapidity of its onset may make early securing of the patency of the airway a lifesaving event. This may occur at the scene, as rescuers have become more sophisticated and better trained to perform endotracheal intubation or, in extreme cases, cricothyroidotomy in the field. Upper airway injury with obstruction can occur in conjunction with lower airway chemical injury and progressive problems with gas exchange, or the upper airway injury may be an isolated event. Patients with upper airway edema may require endotracheal intubation to maintain a patent airway, but as the edema resolves and there is no compromise of gas exchange, such patients can undergo extubation as soon as the airway is patent.

Burn patients often have smoke inhalation as a component of their injury. Smoke inhalation causing inhalation injury combined with burned skin remains the primary cause of death in burn patients.[2] Little progress has been made in reducing mortality in these circumstances.[3] The combination of burned skin and chemical injury to the lower airway by inhaled toxic products of combustion may cause the patient to develop acute respiratory distress syndrome hours or days after the injury.[4] Burning plastic and synthetic fabrics release acroline and other aldehydes, which directly injure the airway mucosa and initiate an inflammatory reaction.[5] Carbon monoxide and cyanide rarely damage the mucosa, but interfere with gas exchange.[6] The need for high volumes of intravenous fluids to resuscitate the patient from their burn injury may create additional pulmonary capillary leakage, which exacerbates the smoke injury problem. This situation develops following the combination of smoke inhalation and burned skin.[7] It usually manifests itself at 24 to 72 hours post injury and is heralded by a falling oxygen saturation. Changes in the chest x-ray often lag behind the development of hypoxia. Many such patients will arrive at the Western Pennsylvania Hospital Burn Center intubated because of the combined injury. Rising mean airway pressures call for sophisticated ventilatory management.

When a prolonged hospital course is anticipated by the need for multiple debridement and skin graft procedures and by the degree of pulmonary dysfunction, a tracheostomy may be indicated. Saffle et al in a randomized study did not find that tracheostomy was associated with earlier weaning from the ventilator nor was it associated with increased survival.[8] Our experience has demonstrated that a tracheostomy provides an easier and more comfortable access to the lower airway than oral or nasal endotracheal intubation. It also allows for easier access to the lower airway for suctioning than oral or nasotrachal intubation. We have had in the past years inadvertent

dislodgment of the endotracheal tube during dressing changes on extensively burned patients. The need to roll the patient from side to side and in some cases to a prone position makes the patient susceptible to dislodgment of the endotracheal tube. With massive facial edema and poor pulmonary function, this can be a fatal complication. The tracheostomy can make dressing changes and wound care safer.

When patients with smoke inhalation and extensive thermal injury to their skin are admitted and endotracheal intubation is found to be necessary, we anticipate the need for prolonged ventilatory support. Such patients in our unit have an elective tracheostomy performed early in their course of treatment. When multiple operations are anticipated and prolonged ventilatory support is anticipated, a tracheostomy provides a safe access to the patient's airway and provides safety during dressing changes and other bedside treatments.

When a tracheostomy is anticipated and the patient has deep partial-thickness or full-thickness burns of the anterior neck, this area of burned skin will be excised and grafted during the course of the patient's first skin graft procedure. The eschar is tangentially excised to viable tissue and a meshed split-thickness skin graft is stapled or sutured in place and oversprayed with fibrin spray tissue glue. Seventy-two hours postgraft, the dressing is changed and the graft take should be uniformly successful (Fig 7–1). Five to 7 days later, the interstices of the graft should be completely epithelialized so that a tracheostomy can be performed through a clean healed wound (Fig 7–2). The survival rate of burn patients with a tracheostomy has improved with attention to grafting neck burns early so that

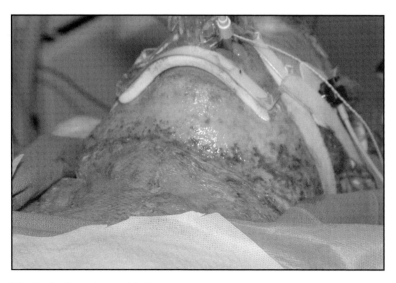

Fig 7–1. A patient with burns to the neck underwent debridement of the burned skin and the application of a meshed, split-thickness skin graft.

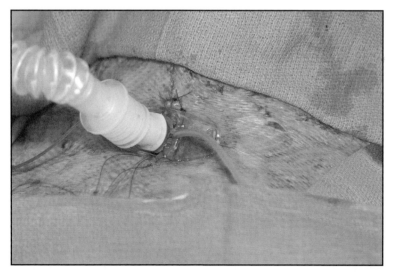

Fig 7–2. The tracheostomy is carried out through the clean, healed wound provided by the skin graft.

tracheostomy can be created through healed clean tissue.[9]

Although we have never done a formal study randomizing patients with the need for ventilatory support to tracheos-tomy or prolonged endotracheal tube intubation, it is our impression that we can be more aggressive with weaning patients who have a tracheostomy from the ventilator because there is no need for reintubation should the patient fail a trial off the ventilator. The ventilator merely may be reconnected.

The need for urgent surgical access to the airway is rare in the experience of burn centers. More and more first responders have the training and ability to perform endotracheal intubation at the scene of fires prior to transfer of the patient to a community hospital or burn center. In extreme cases, cricothyroidotomy can be performed in the field or in the emergency department of a referring hospital. These lifesaving measures are important to master and anyone seeing burn patients at the time of rescue or referral to a community hospital should be prepared to perform these procedures should they become necessary.

Burns of the upper airway and face can cause massive edema. The smoke inhalation can cause upper airway obstruction that makes endotracheal intubation difficult or impossible if such procedures are delayed. Tracheostomy on burn patients should be a well-planned elective surgical procedure. Patients with upper airway edema and/or pulmonary dysfunction requiring ventilatory support, should be intubated well in advance of the need for tracheostomy. Tracheostomy may be performed at the bedside by surgeons familiar with this procedure. Gravvanis et al compared patients who underwent percutaneous tracheostomy in a burn center with patients who underwent a conventional tracheostomy.[10] The authors felt that, in their hands, percutaneous tracheostomy was associated with a lower complication rate and could be performed safely at the bedside. Others have compared bedside versus operating room tracheostomy and found that bedside tracheostomy was lower in charges to the patient. However, the nursing time

and time for assembly of equipment time was not calculated.[11]

The requirements for the safe performance of tracheostomy include an adjustable operating table or bed, excellent lighting, suction, immediately available surgical instruments and tracheostomy cannulas, and adequate help. If an institution can assemble this support at the bedside, a bedside tracheostomy is a reasonable option. We have preferred to perform the tracheostomy on burn patients in the operating room. Many of the patients in our geographic region are obese prior to their burn injury. The burn injury of the upper chest, neck, and head, exacerbates the soft tissue mass of the neck and makes full extension of the neck difficult. We believe this subset of patients do better in an operative room environment than they would with an attempt to create a tracheostomy at the bedside.

It has been our practice over the past 35 years to perform tracheostomy on burn patients in the operating room. The operations are performed by residents at the first-year level with an attending surgeon assisting and present throughout the entirety of the operation. We begin by positioning the patient in an almost seated position with the trunk at at least 45 degrees flexion at the hips. The operation is performed on the operating table rather than the patient's bed so that the surgeon and assistant can be close to the patient without prolonged flexion of their lumbar spines. The upper chest, neck, and face are prepared with the surgeon's choice of antiseptic agent and drapes are placed leaving the patient's face exposed. We find that this allows for easier identification of anatomic landmarks and it allows the anesthetist to observe the progress of the operation.

The burn patient who has a tracheostomy performed often has massive edema of the face and neck. It is our practice to outline anatomic landmarks with a surgical marking pen prior to commencing the operation. The notch in the laryngeal cartilage is identified and marked with a V. The cricothyroid membrane is marked with a horizontal stripe. The extent and position of the vertical incision is then marked with a surgical marker. We use electrodissection beginning with the skin incision and carry this down to the trachea. The thyroid isthimus can be divided with electrocautery or if it is large it can be clamped and suture ligated with absorbable suture material. When the trachea is identified at its junction with the larynx, it is grasped with a small sharp unbent towel clip. This allows a secure grasp of the trachea and it may be pulled anterior and cephalad to expose the area of the second and third tracheal cartilages. The trachea slopes from anterior to posterior as it progresses from cephalad to caudad. The trachea is exposed in its most superior and superficial portion and elevated with the towel clip. Additional soft tissue caudad to the upper part of the trachea is divided with electrocautery.

In teenagers and young adults, a window of tracheal tissue is removed between the second and third cartilages. This window is approximately the size of the desired tracheostomy device. When the window is removed, the anesthetist is asked to pull back the endotracheal tube until it has cleared the window. This allows for immediate readvancement of the endotracheal tube into the trachea should there be a problem with bleeding or access to the lumen. The tracheostomy cannula is then inserted and connected to the anesthesia delivery system.

When end-tidal carbon dioxide and adequate oxygenation and adequate ventilation are confirmed, the endotracheal tube can be removed. A final check of hemostasis is then made to be sure that there is no new bleeding caused by the insertion of the tracheostomy cannula. We have found the use of fibrin tissue glue to be very helpful if there is persistent oozing after the tracheostomy cannula is inserted.

The neck plate on the tracheostomy cannula is then sutured to the skin with 4 stout nonabsorbable nylon or Prolene sutures. The tracheostomy collar is then secured behind the patient's neck and attached to the appropriate openings on the neck plate. When there is no collar, the twill ribbons that come with the tracheostomy cannula are secured. We then place a precut tracheostomy dressing or we place a 4×8 gauze under the neck plate of the tracheostomy device in a U-shaped pattern so that this can apply additional pressure to the operative area. The operation is then terminated.

When the tracheostomy is no longer needed, a cannula can be downsized to size 4 and then removed several days later. Alternatively, we have usually removed the size 8 cannula without downsizing. Patients with and without skin grafts or burns to the anterior neck have uniformly healed without the need for revision of the tracheostomy wounds.

The close supervision of surgical residents and the adherence to the protocol above has resulted in no need for transfusion or returning patients to the operating room for posttracheostomy bleeding. There has been no dislodgment of a tracheostomy tube in the past 35 years, and in follow-up of patients for 12 to 24 months, there have been no complications related to tracheostomy.

REFERENCES

1. Pitt RM, Parker JC, Jurkovich GJ, Taylor AE, Curreri PW. Analysis of altered capillary pressure and permeability after thermal injury. *J Surg Res.* 1987; 42:693-702.
2. Herndon DN, Thompson PB, Traber DL, Abston S. Pulmonary injury in burned patients. *Crit Care Clin.* 1985;1:79-96.
3. Sobel JB, Goldfarb, IW, Slater H, Hammell EJ. Inhalation injury: a decade without progress. *J Burn Care Rehabil.* 1992; 12:573-575.
4. Enkhbaatar P, Traber DL. Pathophysiology of acute lung injury in combined burn and smoke inhalation injury. *Clin Sci.* 2004;107(2):137-143.
5. Birky MM, Clarke FB. Inhalation of toxic products from fires. *Bull NY ACAP Med.* 1981;57:997-1013.
6. Prien T, Traber DL. Toxic compounds and inhalation injury—a review. *Burns.* 1988;14:451-460.
7. Wright MJ, Murphy JT. Smoke inhalation enhances early leukocyte responsiveness to endotoxin. *J Trauma.* 2005;59(1): 64-70.
8. Saffle JR, Morris SE, Edelman L. Early tracheostomy does not improve outcome in burn patients. *J Burn Care Rehabil.* 2002;23(6):431-438.
9. Clark WR, Bonaventura M, Myers W, Kellman R. Smoke inhalation and airway management at a regional burn unit: 1974-1983. II. Airway management. *J Burn Care Rehabil.* 1990;11(2)121-134.
10. Gravvanis AI, Tsoutsos DA, Iconomou TG, Papadopoulos SG. Percutaneous versus conventional tracheostomy in burned patients with inhalation injury. *World J Surg.* 2005;29(12):1571-1575.
11. Lujan HJ, Dries DJ, Gamelli RL. Comparative analysis of bedside and operating room tracheostomies in critically ill patients with burns. *J Burn Care Rehabil.* 1995;16:258-261.

CHAPTER 8

Tracheostomy in Patients with the Obstructive Sleep Apnea Syndrome

JONAS T. JOHNSON

Tracheostomy was an established effective treatment in the management of severe obstructive sleep apnea before positive pressure, bariatric surgery, or other surgical interventions were popularized.[1-4] Over the years, the tracheostomy has maintained an important place in the armamentarium of surgeons who deal with patients with severe obstructive sleep apnea.

Tracheostomy in the treatment of obstructive sleep apnea is a considerable challenge for three basic reasons. First, a tracheostomy may be planned as an intermediate or long-term intervention.

Accordingly, it is ideal to "mature" the stoma by suturing the skin to the mucosa of the trachea. When properly accomplished, this facilitates hygiene and makes tube changing far easier and safer.

The second issue has to do with the difficulty of performing surgery in the morbidly obese. Because of the size of these patients, just getting them to the operating room and onto the operating table is a challenge. Establishment of an anesthetic as well as all the steps in the procedure may be difficult even for the most accomplished and experienced surgeon. Last, the caliber of the neck and the relationship of the soft tissues to the airway vary dramatically in the morbidly obese patients. Most "standard" tracheostomy tubes fit poorly or not at all.

PATIENT SELECTION

Prior to intervention for obstructive sleep apnea, all patients should have a trial of treatment with positive pressure such as CPAP (continuous positive airway pressure). A variety of masks and respiration systems are available. Most patients would agree with the dictum that every effort should be made to establish an alternative effective therapy before tracheostomy is settled on as a solution for obstructive sleep apnea.

The surgeon is advised to carefully evaluate the patient's history as well as the results of a monitored sleep study before embarking on the tracheostomy as a solution for the patient's sleep disorder. Presently, there are 84 distinct sleep disorders listed in the International Classification of Sleep Disorders (ICSD) by the American Sleep Disorders Association.[5] Obstructive sleep apnea syndrome is not the most common sleep disorder. Whereas it is readily apparent that a tracheostomy has the potential to completely relieve upper airway obstruction during sleep, it should be equally apparent that a tracheostomy applied to a patient with a nonobstructive sleep disorder will not be beneficial to the patient.

In general, a tracheostomy is offered only to patients with severe obstructive sleep apnea (apnea-hypoxia indices in excess of 40 events/hour) in whom positive pressure therapy and other surgical therapies have failed. Patients who voice difficulty in initiating and sustaining sleep should be carefully evaluated for other parasomnia or dyssomnia as much as difficulties in initiating or maintaining sleep which suggests a more complex diagnosis than obstructive sleep apnea.

Tracheostomy may be used as a "temporary" intervention adjuvant to other surgical interventions for obstructive sleep apnea in patients with severe symptoms and associated comorbidities such as desaturation-related cardiac arrhythmia and congestive heart failure. This may be especially appropriate when patients can be reliably predicted to be noncompliant with positive pressure during the perioperative period.

In general, tracheostomy is highly effective in relieving apnea entirely in properly diagnosed patients. Accordingly, as a single procedure, it is suitable for patients with severe symptomatic obstructive sleep apnea. Inasmuch as most patients are reluctant to accept tracheostomy as a permanent (lifelong) intervention, many will request that adjunct procedures be accomplished in the hope that tracheostomy can be reversed at some point in the future. We have observed that this may be a reasonable goal in patients who are willing to undergo maxillomandibular advancement with uvulopalatopharyngoplasty or in the group of patients with morbid obesity who achieve major (>125 lbs) weight loss following bariatric surgery.

In either circumstance, it is recommended that the response to surgical intervention be documented objectively with a monitored sleep study prior to decannulation. This can be accomplished by instructing the laboratory to perform the polysomnography with the tracheostomy occluded with a tracheal plug.[6] The patient can, of course, assess independently relief of symptoms by sleeping several nights in a row at home with the tracheostomy plugged.

SURGICAL TECHNIQUE

A tracheostomy in the morbidly obese is technically difficult and rarely accomplished quickly. Given the risk of sedation in this patient population, procedures ideally should be accomplished during general endotracheal anesthesia to establish a stable airway intraoperatively.

Prior to surgery, it is essential that the surgeon address personally his assessment of the patient's airway. Do the temporomandibular joints have full range of motion? Can the neck be extended? Massive obesity may challenge even very experienced anesthesiologists. Flexible fiberoptic endoscopy with awake intubation under topical anesthesia may be an appropriate choice for many patients.

After a general endotracheal anesthesia has been established, the patient should be placed in the supine position. Neck extension is frequently impossible. Cervical landmarks are difficult to palpate. We begin with a reasonably long (4–6 cm) transverse incision intended to overlie the cricoid cartilage. Skin flaps are elevated down to the level of the strap muscles both inferiorly and superiorly. Subsequent to this, the skin flaps are defatted with care being taken to ligate the anterior jugular veins.

Subsequently the strap muscles are separated in the midline and the thyroid isthmus is divided and oversewn. One technique to afford added length for mucocutaneous approximation is to develop an inferiorly based flap from the third and the fourth tracheal rings, which can be sutured directly to the cervical skin. Advancement of rotation flaps to allow circumferential maturation of the stoma is frequently made more complex by the thickness of the skin and the depth of the trachea. Nevertheless, muco-cutaneous approximation without tension on the skin flaps will greatly facilitate postoperative care.[7]

The ideal tracheostomy tube for the perioperative period has an inner cannula (Fig 8-1). The requirement for a rigid inner cannula requires that the tracheostomy tube must always be in the arc of a circle, which, unfortunately, rarely "fits" the shape of the neck especially in this patient population. Attempts to develop a flexible tube with an inner cannula have proven difficult because of problems attaching the flexible portion of the tube to the 15-mm connector. These problems have been addressed at the time of this writing and long tubes with flexible inner cannula are available. Tracheostomy tubes without an inner cannula may be difficult to suction and clean postoperatively. Mucous plugs in the tracheostomy tube may be life threatening.

Tubes without a fixed flange may be difficult to position and may move relative to the position of the patient and his trachea. When tubes are placed too far into the trachea, obstruction of the main stem bronchus may occur. Conversely,

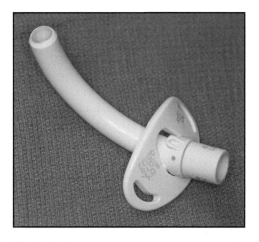

Fig 8–1. Standard tracheostomy tube with an inner cannula. Curve is the arc of a circle.

tubes that are inadequately inserted may be extruded and difficult or impossible to reinsert.

COMPLICATIONS

Sudden relief of long-standing airway obstruction may lead to acute postobstructive pulmonary edema. The best treatment is early identification and positive pressure (positive end expiratory pressure—PEEP).[8]

Failure to have a properly sized tube fixed securely may lead to accidental decannulation or intubation of a single bronchus. An alert, well-trained nursing staff can be a lifesaver.

Bleeding immediately after tracheostomy may suggest inadequate hemostasis. This requires immediate intervention. Hemoptysis weeks or months after surgery is usually an indication of inadequate humidification with resultant tracheitis and crusting. Diagnosis is established with flexible endoscopy. Treatment requires installation of saline and a brief course of broad-spectrum antibiotics. The chronic presence of a foreign body (the tracheostomy tube) may result in formation of granulation of tissue. This friable tissue may bleed and/or obstruct the airway. Removal is often required with a CO_2 laser under local anesthesia.

All tracheostomies are colonized by skin bacteria with *Pseudomonas* being the predominate species. The best care is cleaning the skin, gentle suction, and tube changes when they become crusted. Cellulitis is unusual but may occur. Antibiotics are indicated for cellulitis, but should not be routinely employed for tracheostomy as they select for resistant organisms.

ROUTINE CARE

Breathing through a tracheostomy tube exposes the lower airway to potential pathogens, foreign bodies, and the deleterious effects of inadequately warmed and humidified air. Most patients require daily installation of normal saline. This is available through most drug stores as "saline bullets," which are unit dosed with 5 cc of normal saline. An alternative approach is to have patients make their own normal saline (2 teaspoons of salt in 2 cups of tap water). Unfortunately, this solution is subject to bacterial overgrowth which requires it be mixed daily and the residual from the day's saline be discarded. Individual room humidification with a vaporizer is appropriate in the bedroom while sleeping. The usual home humidifiers do not provide maximum humidification.

Patients with a tracheostomy for obstructive sleep apnea can plug the tracheostomy tube while awake (Fig 8–2). This, of course, allows them to function reasonably normally. The voice is restored to normal and the patient can have a relatively good quality of life.

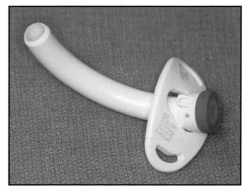

Fig 8–2. Standard tracheostomy tube with plug in place. This allows normal breathing and voice.

Patients should, of course, be warned about the potential dangers of unrestricted water. Clearly, the patient with a tracheostomy tube cannot swim. The potential dangers of work or play on the waterfront or in a boat are evident.

CHOICE OF TRACHEOSTOMY TUBES

A tracheostomy tube is required to maintain the lumen of the tracheostomy. Some authors have advocated for a skin-lined fenestra.[7] Our personal experience is that these procedures eventually fail with tracheal stoma stenosis or, alternatively, they are too wide, which does not allow voicing.

Accordingly, we maintain patients with some form of a lumen keeper. Standard tracheostomy tubes are easy to fix to the neck. Additionally, they are easy to clean and change. Unfortunately, they are unsightly and the projection of the inner cannula can be a nuisance. The alternative is to install a single lumen vent with an attached plug (Figs 8-3A, 8-3B, and 8-3C), which are commercially available. It requires that the surgeon accurately measure the diameter of the tracheostomy site as well as the distance between the skin and the mucosa to afford a proper

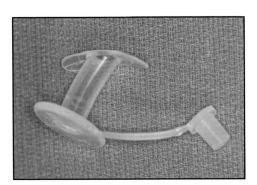

A.

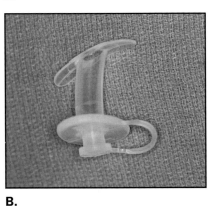

B.

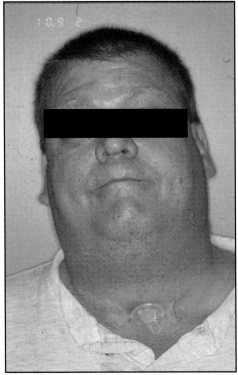

C.

Fig 8–3. A. Hood stoma vent is retained in stoma with inner and outer flanges. **B.** Stoma vent with plug in place for voicing. **C.** Stoma vent in place. Plug introduced during waking hours. Plug removed while sleeping.

fit. The inner flange may occasionally be associated with a granuloma. Additionally, a forceful cough occasionally results in the sudden and explosive displacement of the apparatus. Accordingly they are not suitable for all candidates.

SUMMARY

Tracheostomy can be both a lifesaving and a life-changing experience for the patient with severely symptomatic obstructive sleep apnea. Our experience has been that approximately one-half of the patients accommodate to these tubes and live "happily ever after" requiring intermittent tube changes, excision of granulation tissue, and treatment for tracheitis.

The other half of the patients aspire to get rid of their tubes. This requires further intervention in the form of either the surgery to improve their airways such as maxillomandibular advancement or successful bariatric surgery.

REFERENCES

1. Kuhlo W, Doll E, Franck MC. Successful management of Pickwickian syndrome using long-term tracheostomy. *Dtsch Med Wochenshr.* 1969;94:1286–1290.
2. Tilkian AG, Guilleminault C, Schroeder JS, et al. Sleep-induced apnea syndrome: prevalence of cardiac arrhythmias and their reversal after tracheostomy. *Am J Med.* 1977;63;348–358.
3. Motta J, Guilleminault C, Schroeder JS, Dement WC. Tracheostomy and hemodynamic changes in sleep-inducing apnea. *Ann Intern Med.* 1978:89;454–458.
4. Guilleminault C, Simmons FB, Motta J, et al. Obstructive sleep apnea syndrome and tracheostomy: long-term follow up experience. *Arch Intern Med.* 1981;141: 985–988.
5. American Academy of Sleep Medicine. *International Classification of Sleep Disorders: Diagnostic and Coding Manual*, 2nd ed. Rochester, Minn: Author; 2005.
6. Kim SH, Eisele DW, Smith PL, Schneider H, Schwartz AR. Evaluation of patients with sleep apnea after tracheostomy. *Arch Otolaryngol Head Neck Surg.* 1998; 124(9):996–1000.
7. Campanini A, DeVito A, Frassineti S, Vicini C:.Role of skin-lined tracheostomy in obstructive sleep apnoea syndrome: personal experience. *Acta Otorhinolaryngol Ital.* 2004; 24(2):68–74.
8. Burke AJ, Duke SG, Clyne S, Khoury SA, Chiles C, Matthews BL. Incidence of pulmonary edema after tracheostomy for obstructive sleep apnea. *Otolaryngol Head Neck Surg.* 2001; 125(4):319–323.

CHAPTER 9

Nursing Management of the Patient with a Tracheostomy

MARILYN HUDAK
MARGARET M. HICKEY

Caring for a patient with a tracheostomy requires the coordination of a multidisciplinary team of skilled health care professionals. The health care team must be inclusive and collaborative as a tracheostomy will impact a patient's respiratory system, communication, swallowing, and body image. Nurses are vital to the coordination of the needed consults based on the individual patient's health care needs. Members of this multidisciplinary health care team include the surgeon and other specialty physicians; nurses practicing inpatient, clinic, and home care; respiratory therapists; speech and swallow therapists; clinical dieticians; and social workers. Preparation of the patient and his or her significant other for the operative procedure and after care should begin as soon as the decision to perform the tracheostomy has been made.

PREOPERATIVE MANAGEMENT

A tracheotomy and tracheostomy are two terms that are often used interchangeably. A "tracheotomy" is a surgical incision into the trachea and a "tracheostomy" refers to the actual opening into the trachea, or stoma.[1]

The need for a tracheostomy can be divided into three general categories: (1) to bypass obstruction of the upper airway, (2) to provide a method of removing retained tracheal secretions, and (3) to provide a means of ventilator support. The most common reason today for a tracheostomy is to provide long-term access to the airway in patients who are in need of mechanical ventilation.[2] Other indications for performing a tracheostomy include severe neck or oral injuries, obstructive lesions, postoperative edema or surgical alterations, sleep apnea related to obstruction from obesity, congenital abnormality of the larynx or trachea, inhalation injuries, foreign body, vocal cord paralysis that affects swallowing and causes aspiration, inability to clear secretions, tracheal stenosis, or malacia.[3]

A tracheostomy may be performed as an emergency procedure such as in a trauma or a medical emergency situation; it could be an elective procedure to prevent postoperative airway compromise due to surgical changes or postoperative edema; to provide a route for long-term mechanical ventilation; or to manage obstructive sleep apnea.[4] Unless a tracheostomy is done as an emergency procedure, it is usually performed as a scheduled surgical procedure in the operating room. The tracheostomy may be performed under local or general anesthesia, depending on the patient's medical condition and the surgeon's preference.

Assessment

A preoperative assessment should include a complete history and a physical examination. Question the patient about his or her past medical and surgical history. Determine the patient's compliance with the management of coexisting conditions or past medical problems. Patients tend to pursue the same behavior with all medical conditions and knowledge of past compliance will aid in anticipating the extent of compliance with the current medical situation. Inquire regarding all medications the patient is currently taking including prescription and over-the-counter medications, vitamins, and herbal supplements. A number of over-the-counter and vitamin supplements can affect blood clotting; for example, aspirin may hinder platelet aggregation, and garlic, gingko biloba, and other herbal supplements can prolong bleeding time.[5] Identify any allergies to in-halants, medications, or latex. Inquire in a nonjudgmental manner about the patient's tobacco, alcohol, and other substance use. Alcohol and tobacco use are risk factors for head and neck cancers. Often patients are unwilling to provide an accurate estimate of alcohol consumption and an intentionally high estimate may yield more accurate information.[6] If alcohol use is regular, a plan to prevent withdrawal symptoms may need to be initiated. Assistance and referral to a tobacco cessation and alcohol rehabilitation program to follow the acute hospitalization period should be implemented as appropriate.

Completing a history on a patient prior to tracheostomy is similar to completing a general patient history. It should include information about the chief complaint including a description of the problem in the patient's or significant other's own words. It helps to inquire what changes the patient or significant others noticed leading to the decision to seek medical attention. These may include difficulty breathing or shortness of breath, a change in the voice, a change in eating habits, pain, aspiration on swallowing, or cough. When did the patient first notice these changes? How severe are the symptoms? What has the patient done to alleviate the symptoms? Have these measures helped? Using a process of active listening which repeats and verifies clinical information helps to ensure the history is accurate and will increase the patient's and significant other's trust in the health care provider.[7] The patient should be observed for signs of airway distress or obstruction, such as dyspnea, increased mucus production, ineffective cough, stridor, restlessness, poor oxygenation as per blood gas or pulse oximetry values, suprasternal retraction, and cyanosis.

Preoperative Teaching

Once the decision to perform a tracheostomy has been made, the preoperative teaching should be initiated. This should be unhurried and should take place in a private area. Ideally, preoperative teaching should include the patient and a significant other. The normal airway should be described to the patient, and a thorough explanation of the rationale for the tracheostomy and any other planned surgical alterations given. Diagrams or models are excellent tools to illustrate the normal airway and compare it to the airway alteration after the tracheostomy. If appropriate, depict the changes that have occurred because of the disease process.

Referrals

Preoperative referrals will provide the patient and significant other with an opportunity to discuss concerns and identify problems that may arise during the perioperative period. The patient who will undergo a tracheostomy should consult with a social worker, speech and swallow therapist, and clinical dietician. In meeting with these health care professionals preoperatively, an appropriate plan can be made with the patient and the significant other for surgery and postoperative care including hospitalization, rehabilitation, and home care.

Communication

The patient's ability to speak normally is altered after a trachesotomy. Once a temporary tracheostomy has been performed, the air enters the surgical opening below the vocal cords and thereby bypasses the upper airway. In a patient who has had a permanent tracheostomy or total laryngectomy, the vocal cords are removed, and the trachea is sutured to the skin of the neck. In either case, a communication plan is a key element of the preoperative planning and teaching.

An understanding of why the patient will be unable to speak should be reviewed with both patient and significant other prior to surgery. Alternative methods of communication should be introduced and practiced prior to the time they are needed. Together with the patient and significant other the appropriate communication technique should be selected for the immediate perioperative period.

If the patient is able to read and write, a peel-back dry-erase board (magic slate), dry-erase board and marker, or paper and pencil may be used. If the patient cannot read or write alternative techniques such as flash cards or a communication board can be used. Consultation with the speech and swallow therapist during this preoperative teaching period is helpful as speech and swallowing rehabilitation is a large part of the perioperative care. Consulting the speech and swallow therapist early provides an opportunity for discussion and review of the voice rehabilitation options such as electrolarynx devices, speaking tracheostomy tubes, or tracheosesophageal shunts. This consult will be especially helpful in establishing the perioperative communication plan particularly for those patients with vision or hearing impairments, literacy issues, and language barriers.

Equipment and Procedures

A review of tracheostomy tubes that are commonly used will acquaint the patient and significant other with the tube that will be placed after the surgery. It may help to use a pre-assembled teaching tray containing tracheostomy tubes, suction catheters, humidification devices, and any other equipment that may be used after surgery. This equipment tray gives the patient and family an opportunity to have hands-on experience in a nonthreatening environment. Review the procedures both preoperatively and postoperatively to familiarize the patient and significant other with the hospital routine. These measures will help to minimize preoperative anxiety.

Psychosocial Preparation

Psychosocial counseling is integrated into all aspects of the preoperative preparation. The patient and significant other should be given the opportunity to discuss concerns about the need for a tracheostomy, the resulting changes in communication, changes in physical appearance and body image, social concerns, and financial issues. Counseling

should be performed with the patient and significant other together and separately to assess coping skills. A consult with a social worker at this time can be beneficial in supplying information regarding support groups and addressing financial concerns. An evaluation of the home situation and ability for either the patient or caregiver to provide independent care guides the decision for potential placement in an extended care facility. Referrals should be initiated early in the perioperative course if needed.

POSTOPERATIVE MANAGEMENT

Immediately after surgery the patient should be placed in an area where the nursing staff can provide close monitoring. Whether the setting is an intensive care unit, special care unit, or a general medical-surgical unit, the patient should be in a room close to the nurse's station where the nurse can see and hear the patient. During the immediate postoperative period, the following concerns should be addressed: airway management, wound care, communication, nutrition, and discharge planning. To enable the nurse to provide the necessary care, the room should be equipped with humidified oxygen and tracheostomy mask, suction with sterile tracheal suction catheters and a yankauer or tonsillar suction tips, and an extra tracheostomy tube of the same type and size in case accidental decannulation should occur. There should be an emergency cart nearby.

Postoperatively the patient should be placed in a mid to high Fowler's position. Elevating the head of the bed helps to minimize postoperative edema, increase air exchange, enhance the patient's ability to cough and mobilize secretions, increase the ease of suctioning, and overall promotes the patients general comfort.

Airway Management

A key concept in managing the patient's airway successfully is to understand how to care for the tracheostomy tube. The tracheostomy tube provides an artificial pathway to secure an airway. The tube cannot be managed in isolation. Special considerations need to be given to the patient's special needs. What was the rationale for the tracheostomy tube placement: does the patient require mechanical ventilation; is it to bypass upper airway edema secondary to trauma or a cancer procedure; is it to bypass an airway obstruction; it is a temporary measure, or is it permanent such as in a patient with a total laryngectomy? An understanding of the patient's medical history will guide postoperative decisions and allow an individualized care plan to be developed.

The type of tracheostomy tube used will depend on the physician's preference, institutional guidelines, and the patient's specific needs. A number of different types and models of tracheostomy tubes are available. Tracheostomy tubes can be metal or plastic. Metal tubes are constructed of silver or stainless steel and are not commonly used. Plastic tubes can be made from polyvinyl chloride or silicone. Polyvinyl chloride is thermolabile and softens at body temperature conforming to patient's anatomy. Silicone tubes are naturally soft and unaffected by temperature.[7]

Some tracheostomy tubes have only a single cannula whereas others come with an easily removable inner cannula. The inner cannula, when present, can be removed for cleaning or when it gets blocked with secretions. It is held in place by either a twist lock or pressure clip fitting at the base of the flange. Inner cannulas can be reusable or disposable; disposable cannulas are more often used in hospital settings. Each tube has a faceplate, a lateral neckplate that lies against the patient's skin and helps hold the tracheostomy tube in place. The faceplate has slits through which the tracheostomy ties or a holder can be threaded to fasten the tube around the neck. There are a variety of faceplates. Some faceplates can be flexible and continuous with the tube; others can be made of PVC and swivel in response to patient movement; other tubes may be adjustable so the faceplate can move up or down the length of the tube allowing for adjustments to be made for the individual patient.

Tracheostomy tubes come in a variety of diameters, lengths, and curvatures. For example, the laryngectomy tube, which is used for a patient who has had a total laryngectomy and a permanent stoma, is shorter and less curved than the standard tracheostomy tube. This length and curvature is customized for the location of the laryngectomy stoma, which is placed lower than the tracheostomy stoma.

Tracheostomy tubes can be available with or without a cuff. A cuff is a soft balloon around the distal end of the tube that can be inflated to form a seal between the tracheostomy tube and tracheal wall to help prevent aspiration and/or allow mechanical ventilation in patients with respiratory failure. Today's tracheostomy cuffs are high volume and low pressure. This cuff engineering allows the pressure of the cuff to be distributed across a maximal area of the trachea minimizing the risk of tracheal stenosis. Tracheostomy cuffs can be filled with air, foam, or water. Air-filled low pressure cuffs have pilot balloons and some models are available with safety valves that allow air to be released when the cuff pressure exceeds 20 to 25 mm Hg. Foam cuffs minimize pressure to the tracheal mucosa by employing an open system. The pilot balloon must remain open at all times. This allows air to be displaced from the foam into the atmosphere when pressure rises within the trachea and likewise allows the air to re-enter and the foam to re-expand once the trachea relaxes. For long-term applications, some newer tubes have tight-to-shaft cuffs. This cuff does not add much to the diameter of the tube and can facilitate the tracheostomy tube changes by eliminating the lip that forms when standard cuffs are deflated. This model may be especially useful for children because deflated air can more easily pass around the tube in the trachea allowing for speech.

Fenestrated tracheostomy tubes also are available. Fenestrated tubes have an opening or openings in the outer cannula that permit air to pass from the lungs through the openings in the tracheostomy tube up into the patient's upper airway. This tube is most commonly used for weaning a patient off a tracheostomy tube. It allows the viability of the upper airway to be tested while maintaining airway patency. It also allows the patient to speak, as it permits air to pass through the vocal cords. If a solid inner cannula is inserted, this seals off the fenestration and air cannot pass through the upper airway.

Tracheostomy Care

Caring for a patient with a tracheostomy tube often can be challenging. The key to optimizing care in this special patient population is to understand the basic principles of tracheostomy in the context of the individual's unique situation and needs. The basics of tracheostomy care include clearing the airway or suctioning, cuff management, humidification, cleaning the tube, securing the tube, and wound care.

Maintaining a Patent Airway

Airway maintenance is the first priority in caring for a patient with a tracheostomy. Monitoring the patient's respiratory status is imperative. Careful assessment of the patient's rate, rhythm, and depth of respirations, auscultation of breath sounds in all lung fields, reviewing oxygenation by pulse oximetry or arterial blood gases, and evaluation of the amount, color, and consistency of mucus are all important components of the assessment. Pulmonary toilet needs to be performed regularly; this includes: positioning changes; coughing and deep breathing (if the patient is not ventilator dependent); and suctioning as necessary. Chest physiotherapy and pulmonary treatments may be prescribed to help mobilize secretions.

If a patient is not ventilator-dependent, suctioning should be used when a cough is not sufficient to clear the mucus. The cough is typically weaker in a patient with a tracheostomy tube. It is important to coach the patient to cough and deep breathe. Place the patient in an upright position and instruct him or her to take three deep breaths, followed by a strong cough. The patient should be instructed to use the cough and deep breathing technique every hour while awake to help minimize the risk of pneumonia. Sterile saline may be instilled to help moisten and loosen the bloody secretions present with a fresh tracheostomy and stimulate a strong cough. Assess the patient's breath sounds and the tenacity and character of secretions. Suctioning should be performed if needed to maintain a clear airway. The act of suctioning creates mechanical irritation to the mucosa of the bronchi and, if done unnecessarily, will actually increase mucus production.

Suctioning can be done using sterile or clean technique. It is this authors' belief that health care professionals should use sterile technique; clean technique can be used once the patient is assuming responsibility for the procedure. Each health care institution will have a specific procedure for suctioning but all will include the same basic principles (Table 9–1).

Table 9–1. Suctioning Procedure

Assemble necessary equipment

Sterile gloves

Sterile suction catheter (no larger than half of the lumen of the tracheostomy tube)

Sterile cup

Sterile water

Oxygen, manual resuscitation bag

Source of negative pressure

Procedure

1. Check suction source it should be at –120 to –150 mm Hg with tubing occluded.
2. Wash hands, apply goggles and sterile gloves.
3. Connect suction catheter to source of negative pressure.
4. Fill basin with sterile water.
5. Provide pre-oxygenation by administering oxygen via trach mask and asking the patient to take 3 to 4 deep breaths, using manual resuscitation bag (MRB) connected to 100% oxygen, or adjusting ventilator to deliver 100% oxygen.
6. If secretions are thick, 3 to 5 cc sterile saline may be instilled into the airway.
7. Gently insert suction catheter, without suction. Insert approximately 5 to 6 inches. Stop if obstruction is met.
8. Apply suction intermittently during removal of suction catheter. Use gentle rotating motion while removing catheter.
9. Suction for 5 to 10 seconds.
10. Assess airway and repeat suctioning as necessary.
11. Administer oxygen or use MRB to re-oxygenate.
12. Apply humidified oxygen at prior setting.

Controversy exists over the need to mechanically bag a patient prior to suctioning. Use of the manual resuscitation bag (MRB) may increase the inspiratory volume and help mobilize secretions; however, this also may place undo stress on the surgical anastamosis of a head and neck surgical patient. The authors believe if the patient is able to take deep breaths on their own with oxygen delivered via a tracheostomy mask, they do not need to be hyperventilated with an MRB.

Secretions should be monitored and documented for any change in color, amount, and odor. The patient's vital signs, especially temperature and white blood cell count should be observed for any acute changes that could indicate infection. Breath sounds should be evaluated every 4 to 8 hours. Rales, rhonchi, and wheezing should be reported to the physician.

Humidification

Because the humidification system of the upper airway is bypassed in the patient with a tracheostomy, supplemental humidification is necessary to prevent drying and crusting of the secretions. Patients on a ventilator will receive continuous humidification via the ventilator circuitry. High humidity can be applied to nonventilator patients using a humidified oxygen mist via a tracheostomy collar. Another technique is to instill up to 5 mL of sterile normal saline solution into the tracheostomy tube three to four times daily. This helps to moisten the mucosa, loosen secretions, and stimulate cough.[8] Supplemental moisture can also be provided by placing normal saline solution into an atomizer and spraying the solution into the tracheostomy tube. A normal saline moistened tracheostomy bib, worn over the tracheostomy, helps to add moisture to every inhaled breath. Heat-moisture exchangers are available (Fig 9–1) and can be attached to the end of the tracheostomy tube. This apparatus is most often used for children. Adult sizes may be heavy and cumbersome. Additional humidification can be added to the room using a cold mist humidifier or the patient can sit in a steam-filled bathroom.

Cuff Management

A cuffed tracheostomy tube is generally used in the immediate postoperative period. A cuffed tube helps to minimize aspiration, provide hemostasis by applying pressure to the tracheal wall, and provide an airtight seal for the patient receiving controlled or assisted ventilation.[1] Excessive pressure in a tracheostomy tube cuff can result in damage to

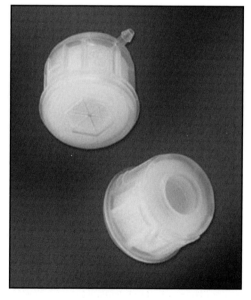

Fig 9–1. Tracheostomy heat moisture exchanger. (Courtesy of Ballard Medical Products.)

the tracheal mucosa resulting in tracheal ischemia and necrosis. The high volume, low pressure cuffed tubes help to minimize pressure but careful monitoring of the intracuff pressure is necessary. Tracheal capillary perfusion pressure is normally 25 to 35 mm Hg. The pressure exerted by the cuff to the tracheal mucosa is thought to be less than the pressure in the cuff; therefore, the maximum intracuff pressure should be 25 mm Hg (34 mm H_2O). If the cuff pressure is too low aspiration may occur, therefore, the recommended cuff pressure should be 20 to 25 mm Hg or (25-35 mm H_2O).[7] Cuff pressure should be monitored regularly using a syringe, stopcock, and manometer (Fig 9–2). This allows the cuff volume to be adjusted simultaneously when the pressure measurement is taken. If the patient does not need a cuffed tube, replacement with an uncuffed tube should be done as soon as possible.

Routine deflation of the cuff is no longer required with the use of low-pressure tracheostomy cuffs; however, cuff deflation is still required to remove secretions that puddle above the tracheostomy cuff. Suction the tracheostomy tube and the patient's mouth to remove secretions that may be aspirated during deflation. The cuff should be deflated during exhalation to prevent aspiration. The patient should then cough or be suctioned while the cuff is deflated so the accumulated secretions can be removed. The cuff should then be reinflated during inspiration. Recently, a tracheostomy tube capable of subglottic suction has been introduced to the market; with this tube the cuff would not need to be deflated to allow removal of secretions.

Care of the Inner Cannula

If the patient's tracheostomy tube has an inner cannula, keeping that cannula clean is imperative. Cleaning the inner cannula should be performed as often as necessary to maintain tube patency. Many tubes are available with a disposable inner cannula that can be discarded after each use. This is a timesaving measure for the hospitalized patient but can become expensive for the patient discharged home with a tracheostomy tube in place. Reusable inner cannulas are available for most tracheostomy tubes. They are cleaned with a diluted solution of half hydrogen peroxide and half normal saline. A tracheostomy or small bottlebrush is helpful in removing dried secretions. The hydrogen peroxide breaks down mucus that can build up and occlude the cannula. Hydrogen peroxide can damage healthy tissue and must be rinsed off thoroughly. The inner cannula should be thoroughly rinsed with water and excess water removed prior to reinserting it into the outer cannula.

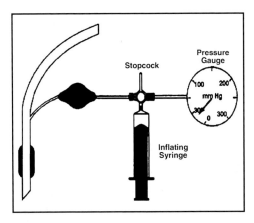

Fig 9–2. Diagram of the equipment used to measure cuff pressure. (Reprinted with permission from: Hess, D. R. Tracheostomy tubes and related appliances. *Respiratory Care*, 50[4]:503.)

Wound Care

The tracheostomy stoma or wound site must be kept clean and dry. The stoma site should be cleaned regularly. Sterile technique should be used when the nurse is providing care to the tracheostomy site. Once the patient is taught the procedure, clean technique may be used. The tracheostomy site and skin under the neck plate of the tracheostomy tube should be cleaned with cotton applicators and half-strength hydrogen peroxide. Hydrogen peroxide helps to remove mucus crusts but it should be rinsed off well and dried. If a tracheostomy dressing is used under the flange or neck plate of the tube, the dressing should be changed when wet or soiled. A moist dressing is a medium for bacterial growth and should be avoided. A tracheostomy dressing, which is precut with a slit to fit around the tube, should be used. If this is not available, a 4×4 gauze dressing can be used but it should be folded and not cut. A cut gauze pad may expose the patient to loose threads that can be inhaled or get twisted around the tracheostomy tube.

Tracheostomy Ties

Following surgery, the tracheostomy tube may be sutured into place, secured with tracheostomy ties made from twill tape, or both. Sutures are usually removed within a few days of surgery and replaced with tracheostomy twill tape ties or a tracheostomy holder. A major complication of tracheostomy is accidental decannulation and keeping the tube securely in place is the first step to avoiding this potential tragedy. It is important to secure the tube well, while maintaining patient comfort by minimizing friction and pressure on the neck. Traditionally,

twill tape was used to secure the tracheostomy tube. It must be tied securely, yet with enough give to enable the nurse to slip one finger under the tape. This will prevent the twill tape from constricting the patient, as the tape does not stretch. Changing twill tape tracheostomy ties usually requires two people: one person must hold the tracheostomy tube in place while a second person threads the tape through the slots on the faceplate and ties it securely. Specialized tracheostomy tube holders are available (Fig 9–3). These holders have a wider diameter than twill tape that helps to distribute pressure and prevent skin irritation. Some models have elastic in the band that allows patient movement while holding the tube securely. Velcro™ is used to secure the tube, making it easier and faster to apply. Regardless of whether twill tape or a tracheostomy tube holder is used, either device must be changed whenever wet or soiled.

Changing the Tracheostomy Tube

Although the technique for changing temporary and permanent tracheostomy tubes is the same, the timing of the initial change is different. The initial changing of a tracheostomy tube is a physician's

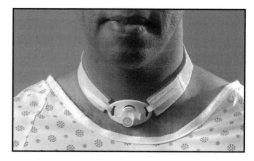

Fig 9–3. Tracheostomy tube holder. (Courtesy of Dale Medical Products.)

responsibility. Future tracheostomy tube changes are a nurse's responsibility but will depend on the individual institution's policy and procedure. A temporary tracheostomy tube is not changed until a tract as formed, usually 5 to 7 days after surgery and is typically done by two nurses who are specially trained in the procedure. A patient should have meals or tube feedings held for at least one hour prior to the tube change to decrease the risk of aspiration. An assessment must always be done immediately after placement of the new tube. Ensure that the patient has a good exchange of air via the tube and that a suction catheter can easily be passed. Assess that the chest rises easily and with equal volume. Ask the patient if they are breathing easily. A permanent tracheostomy (total laryngectomy) tube can be changed anytime postoperatively as the opening is permanent. One nurse can change a permanent tracheostomy tube.

Recognizing and Preventing Accidental Tube Displacement

Accidental displacement of the tracheostomy tube, especially in the first few days following the tracheostomy, can result in a life-threatening emergency. Tracheostomy displacement can lead to respiratory failure. Tracheostomy displacement is a complication in which the tube dislodges from the trachea lumen. Causes of a displaced tracheostomy tube include: a tracheostomy tube which is too short for the patient's neck; patient movement or the patient pulls at the tracheostomy tube due to confusion; excessive forceful coughing; loose tracheostomy ties; a break in sutures; or can occur when changing the tracheostomy tube ties or the tube itself. Signs of a dis-

placed tracheostomy include: no air passing from the tracheostomy tube, inability to pass a suction catheter through the tracheostomy, change in voice quality (stronger voice), a drop in oxygen saturation, and /or stridor.

To decrease the likelihood of the tracheostomy tube being displaced the nurse must take precautions to ensure the ties are secure at all times and special care when changing tracheostomy ties as described earlier in this chapter. Tracheostomy ties that are too tight may cause facial edema due to lack of circulation or cardiac arrhythmias due to pressure on the carotid arteries. Ties that are too loose may allow the tube to move and potential tube displacement resulting in the tube pressing up against the posterior wall of the trachea or into the subcutaneous tissues of the neck.

Patients who require reconstructive surgery and have a free flap to the head and neck cannot have anything restricting over the reconstructed area. Therefore, in these patients the traditional tracheostomy ties will not be used and the tracheostomy tube faceplate will be tacked with sutures on all four corners. Assessment of the integrity of skin holding sutures in place is necessary and any loose or missing sutures should be reported to the physician. The physician should also be notified if the patient is confused and is pulling at the tracheostomy tube; unable to follow restrictions on activity; or has stridor, or bronchospasms with excessive coughing. Additional physician orders such as wrist restraints or breathing treatments would be needed in these cases to decrease chances of tube displacement.

If a tracheostomy tube less than 7 days old becomes displaced, the nurse should immediately notify the physician. If the patient has stay sutures (two 6-inch sutures attached on each side of the trachea, also known as traction sutures) use them to keep the airway open while waiting for help. Often these sutures are labeled in the operating room designating the left and right suture. Pull these sutures apart in the direction marked to lift the trachea up and to open the stoma.[9] Do not cross the sutures or allow them to tangle, as this would close the stoma. A physician should reinsert the tracheostomy tube. Part of tracheostomy care should be ensuring that the stay sutures are separated, labeled as left and right, and maintained in place by tape. This small step in care can be lifesaving should the tracheostomy become displaced. A professional nurse may change a tracheostomy tube after 5 to 7 days as a tract will be formed by this time. This may be dependent on the institution's policy and the nurse should be adequately instructed in the procedure. Table 9–2 outlines the procedure on changing a tracheostomy tube.

Some situations will require immediate intervention to reinstate the airway. The professional nurse must be educated on handling an airway emergency to prevent a respiratory arrest in these situations. If stay sutures have not been used or have been removed and the tube cannot easily be reinserted, the nurse can insert a suction catheter into the stoma to allow for passage of air and serve as a guide for reinsertion of a tube. The tracheostomy tube should be threaded over the suction catheter into the stoma. The suction catheter is then removed and the tube secured. The tracheostomy tube should be easily inserted without resistance. Resistance could indicate the tracheostomy is going into a false passage or track. Have a fiberoptic laryngoscope

ready at the bedside for the physician to ensure the tracheostomy is in the proper place and a tracheostomy tray that includes a pair of tracheal dilators and an extra tracheostomy tube nearby at all times. The professional nurse should ensure that a stat chest x-ray is ordered whenever a tracheostomy is replaced due to displacement. The chest x-ray will confirm the tracheostomy tube is in the proper place and rule out complications associated with a dislodged tube such as mediastinal emphysema or tension pneumothorax. The patient should be closely monitored for further respiratory distress including frequent respiratory assessment and the use of pulse oximetry.

A displaced or obstructed tracheostomy is an emergency that needs quick action to prevent respiratory arrest. Staff must be educated on resuscitation procedures for both a tracheostomy patient and laryngectomy patient and know the anatomic differences. A sign should be placed above the bed and on the front of a chart stating the patient is a laryngectomy patient and to resuscitate via a cuffed tracheostomy tube. A laryngectomy patient must have MRB to tracheostomy tube ventilation during a cardiopulmonary arrest as they have no oral airway. Any patient being bagged via the tracheostomy tube must have an inflated cuffed tube in place. This is necessary to ensure that the air will not escape around the tracheostomy tube and will be delivered to the lungs in sufficient volume.

Decannulation

Decannulation (removal of the tracheostomy tube) may occur once the patient's medical condition resolves and when the patient is able to maintain a patent

Table 9–2. Changing a Tracheostomy Tube

1. Explain the procedure to patient.

2. Wash hands.

3. Wear gloves.

4. Assemble equipment: tracheostomy tube with outer cannula, inner cannula, and obturator; tracheostomy ties; tracheostomy dressing; suction catheter; oxygen; cotton-tipped swabs; hydrogen peroxide; normal saline solution (NSS); water soluble lubricant; scissors; 2 × 2 gauze pads; tracheostomy gauze.

5. If inserting a cuffed tube: inflate cuff to check for leaks then deflate the cuff.

6. Insert tracheostomy ties or Velcro holder into neck flange and obturator into outer cannula.

7. Insert obturator into the outer tracheostomy cannula.

8. Place a small amount of water-soluble lubricant on tip of obturator and tube.

9. Have patient cough to clear airway and suction both tracheal and oral secretions.

10. Deflate patient's tracheostomy cuff if present.

11. Remove in-dwelling tube from patient's stoma by cutting or removing ties.

12. If traction sutures are present: pull the upper suture upward and outward, and pull the lower suture downward and outward to open the stoma. If not present place a shoulder roll beneath the scapula to help extend the neck and open the airway.

13. Clean the stoma with hydrogen peroxide and water to remove crusts; wipe with cotton-tipped applicator soaked with NSS (use care not to let solution run into trachea) and pat dry with 2 × 2 gauze.

14. Instruct the patient to take a deep breath and insert tube gently, using obturator to guide tube into trachea.

15. Immediately remove obturator.

16. Tie tracheostomy tube securely, allowing one finger to be inserted between tie and skin of neck.

17. Reinflate cuff if present.

18. Insert disposable or reusable inner cannula.

19. Tape stay sutures (if present) in place and label as left and right.

20. Place tracheostomy gauze under neck flange of outer cannula.

21. Assess for ease of breathing and ability to easily pass a suction catheter.

22. Deliver humidified air/oxygen via tracheostomy mask.

airway. Once the decision is made to remove the tracheostomy tube, several steps need to be taken before determining if the patient can tolerate the absence of the tracheostomy tube. First, the patient must be able to manage their secretions. This is evaluated by a patient's ability to tolerate the cuff deflated without evidence of aspiration. The patient must also demonstrate an adequate cough and no longer have a need for mechanical ventilation.

The tracheostomy tube may be removed quickly or by a weaning process. Patients who are appropriate for rapid removal of the tracheostomy tube would be those who have very little or no upper airway edema, have a strong cough, and have no risk of rapid physical deterioration related to comorbitities. A second method is to use the downsizing approach or the use of a fenestrated tube. The tracheostomy tube is downsized to a smaller uncuffed tube that allows air to pass around the tracheostomy tube and through the upper airway or a fenestrated tracheostomy tube is placed which allows the air to pass through the fenestrated openings of the tube. A cap is then applied to the tracheostomy tube opening. This blocks all air from passing through the tube and forces expired air to pass either around the downsized tube or through the fenestrated tube into the upper airway. This will allow the patient to speak. Using a fenestrated tube or downsizing the tube allows both for emergency airway access and continued suctioning as needed. The use of a smaller tube reduces discomfort, may facilitate swallowing, and poses less risk for development of airway lesions compared to the presence of a full-size tracheostomy tube.[10]

Patients that tolerate a capped tracheostomy tube for 24 hours may be decan-nulated. Patients may be monitored with pulse oximetry for at least 24 hours after decannulation. Nurses should report any sustained oxygen saturation below 90%, stridor, or signs of aspiration. All suction equipment, and a tracheostomy tube of equal and one size smaller than what was removed should be maintained at the bedside in case the tracheostomy tube needs to be reinserted. Emergency equipment needs to be readily available such as a tracheostomy tray, oxygen, manual resuscitation bag, varying sizes of tracheostomy and endotracheal tubes, and a flexible laryngoscope.

Following removal of the tracheostomy tube, the skin edges are approximated with tape or adhesive strips and an occlusive airtight dressing is applied over the stoma (Fig 9–4). The patient is instructed to apply pressure to the stoma covering when speaking, swallowing, or coughing to prevent the escape of air and secretions and promote healing. Table 9–3 outlines the process to apply an occlusive stoma dressing. This dressing needs to be changed whenever it becomes wet or soiled. Dressing changes may need to be done often, especially after meals in the first 24 hours after decannulation. As time passes the stoma begins to heal and the frequency of the dressing change diminishes.

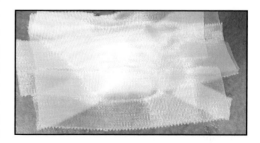

Fig 9–4. Occlusive dressing at tracheotomy site.

Table 9–3. Stoma Dressing Instructions

1. Wash hands and wear gloves.
2. Gently clean stoma with half strength peroxide and water with a 2 × 2 gauze.
3. Pat dry with 2 × 2 gauze pad.
4. Commercial products may be used to increase tape adhesion, such as SKIN-PREP™; do not apply directly over opening, and allow to dry completely.
5. Cut 3 pieces of half-inch clear 3M Transpore™ tape approximately 2.5 inches long. Split tape down to middle to make three ¼-inch strips (discard remaining pieces).
6. Pull edges of stoma together and apply clear tape in an "X" fashion. Use third piece of tape to go across the center.
7. Cut 3 inches of clear half-inch 3M Transpore™ tape approximately 3 inches in length and set aside.
8. Fold a 2 × 2 gauze pad, fold it in half, and apply directly over the middle of the stoma.
9. Cover the 2 × 2 gauze pad with the 3 pieces of cut tape at the top, middle, and bottom to make an occlusive dressing.
10. Educate the patient on the need to hold and press on the 2 × 2 gauze pad when speaking or coughing. Change dressing only when wet as excessive changes can lead to skin breakdown.

Communication

Patients with a tracheostomy often can experience difficulty communicating with family and the health care team. It is the nurse's responsibility to ensure an appropriate means of communication is made available so the patient can effectively express their physical and psychological needs.

Nonverbal behaviors such as mouthing words, gestures, writing, and head nods are the principal means of communication used by temporarily voiceless adults.[11] Communication between patients and caregivers may end up being limited in the form of yes/no questions or simple commands. Tools such as pen and paper, alphabet/picture board, erase board, or augmentative and alternative communi-

cation devices should be available. Although these methods work for many patients, it may be a challenge for patients who are sedated; are experiencing pain; have limited mobility; are visually impaired; or have limited literacy or language barriers. These factors add to the complexity of communication during the recovery period.

One device that can be used to enhance communication is a one-way speaking valve that can be placed on the distal end of the tracheostomy tube to allow exhaled air to be forced around an uncuffed tube or through an uncuffed fenestrated tube (Fig 9–5). This device can improve the quality of voice that can be obtained by using a fenestrated tube alone. Be sure that if using a fenestrated tracheostomy tube with an inner can-

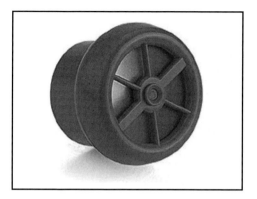

Fig 9–5. One-way speaking valve. (Courtesy of Passy-Muir, Inc.)

nula, the inner cannula is fenestrated as well. The one-way speaking valve allows the patient to breathe in through the tracheostomy tube and inhibits expiration through the tube forcing the expired air up around or through the fenestrated openings of the tracheostomy tube. This allows the exhaled air to vibrate the vocal cords of the patient with a temporary tracheostomy. The one-way speaking valve should not be used with an inflated cuff on a temporary tracheostomy tube or with the patient who has had a total laryngectomy. This would result in obstructing the patient's airway. For safety reasons, patients who are capable should always be taught how to remove a one-way speaking valve in case of respiratory distress and instructed to notify the nurse. Educate the patient not to wear the valve during sleep. A sign should be placed above the patient's bed, on the tracheostomy tube, and on the front of the chart warning staff about precautions with a one-way speaking valve.

An electrolarynx can be provided to permit verbal communication. An intraoral adaptor for the electrolarynx may be used for patients who cannot place pressure on the neck related to healing of a surgical site. Esophageal speech also can be used. Air is forced into the top of the esophagus and expelled through the mouth. This air movement will vibrate the walls of the esophagus and create the "sound" of voice. This technique is often difficult to master and has been augmented by a surgical procedure called a tracheal-esophageal puncture (TEP). The TEP is a surgically created opening from the trachea into the esophagus. Once this tract is healed a one-way valve can be inserted which permits air to flow from the trachea into the esophagus while preventing transportation of food or liquids from the esophagus into the trachea. With the one-way speaking valve inserted, the patient occludes the end forcing the air to enter the esophagus supplementing esophageal speech.

Computer devices such as augmentive and alternative communication (AAC), and electronic voice output communication aids (VOCAs), are in early stages of study as to their effectiveness for a variety of voiceless postoperative patients (Fig 9–6). VOCAs combine synthesized, or prerecorded, digitalized speech with picture icons or message buttons, which help hospitalized patients audibly, communicate with caregivers and visitors.[11] Whatever method of communication is used, whether it is a pencil and paper or advanced computer technology it must be assessed for its effectiveness by the patient, family, nurse, and speech and swallow therapist.

Patients unable to speak should be given extra time to communicate. The nurse should not "second guess" what the patient is trying to say. This time can be used to observe the patient for nonverbal cues that reflect need for nursing intervention such as airway patency, anxiety, or pain. Nurses should ensure the

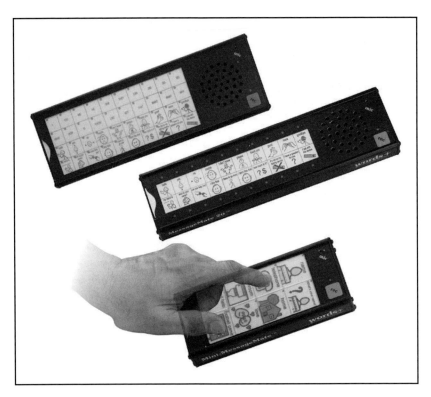

Fig 9–6. Augmentive and alternative communication device—Message-mate model. (Courtesy of Words+.)

patient's call bell is always within reach. A nurse call bell is a voiceless patient's life line, as they cannot call out for an emergency. The call bell can be looped around a side rail or it can be secured with a safety pin to the patient's hospital gown. It is reassuring for speechless patients to know that they will be helped quickly. A note should be attached to the main call light system at the central nursing station that informs the staff if the patient is unable to speak as unit secretaries often respond to patients via the intercom system. When a speechless patient is expected to answer to an intercom voice, the patient's anxiety often escalates.

On specialized units catering to tracheostomy patients, it may be prudent to disable the call light system so the bell can only be turned off inside the patient's room once it is answered. Patients who are incapable of using a call bell and who cannot speak should be placed next to the nurse's station for close observation and should be monitored with pulse oximetry. There are sensitive-to-touch call lights available for patients with extremely limited mobility. Any slight pressure such as a turn of the head will cause an alarm bell for the nurse. Such call bells are typically pinned to the pillow. Every effort by the nurse must be made to ensure that nonsocial patients have a way to communicate for help.

Consultation with the speech and swallow therapist starts at the preoperative stage and is continued throughout hospitalization. The nurse should observe the consultation with the speech and swallow therapist to reinforce any instructions provided. Time should be scheduled for the significant others to meet with the speech therapist. Having effective communication will decrease anxiety, allow patients to express their physical and emotional needs and participate in care, and facilitate teaching and a timely discharge home. A speech and swallow therapist will continue to follow and evaluate patients at home via home health agencies or in the outpatient setting.

Nutrition

Swallowing may be impaired due to the presence of a tracheostomy tube that may impact the patient's nutritional intake. A tracheostomy tube tethers the larynx and prevents it from elevating to allow normal airway protection by the epiglottis. Many studies have demonstrated that patients are at a significantly increased risk for aspiration when a tracheostomy is in place.[10] Aspiration is defined as the passage of material below the level of the vocal folds into the trachea, which may cause marked pulmonary dysfunction.[12] Caution should be exercised before initiating oral feedings in a patient with a tracheostomy and should not be started without a physician's order. If at any time the nurse suspects the patient is aspirating, the nurse should stop feedings and notify the physician. Expert nursing skills play an important role in early recognition of aspiration.

Prior to oral feedings, the patient is best assessed by a speech and swallow therapist for the ability to swallow without aspirating. The therapist can identify the appropriate food consistencies, swal-

lowing techniques, and patient positioning to aid in the swallowing process. Liquids move through the phases of swallowing quickly and may be easily aspirated secondary to any alteration in the swallowing phases, discomfort from the surgical procedure, or tethering of the larynx by the tracheostomy tube. Honorable pureed foods may be more easily tolerated because of the patient's ability to actively manipulate the food bolus thus decreasing possible aspiration. A barium swallow may be ordered to visualize the patient's swallowing abilities and aspiration risk. If aspiration occurs during swallowing, the patient may require enterable feedings until the risk for aspiration subsides. If the patient is able to eat by mouth, instruct them to eat in a sitting position and to remain in the upright position for 1 to 2 hours after meals. If a cuffed tracheostomy tube is in place, the cuff should be inflated during meals and for at least 1 hour after eating. These measures help to minimize aspiration during swallowing as well as prevent potential aspiration of any subsequent gastric reflux. A proton-pump inhibitor agent may be prescribed to decrease acid reflux. Regardless of the route of nutrition, consultation with a dietitian for a baseline assessment and monitoring of the patient's weight and caloric intake is advisable. The dietician can develop the appropriate diet and nutritional supplements needed to ensure adequate caloric and nutritional intake that is vital to the healing process.

Nursing duties related to nutrition include: monitoring of the patient's weight, nutritional intake, swallowing ability, and diet tolerance. The nurse should assess for any pain, nausea, and/or vomiting, constipation, or diarrhea. Reviewing the dietary plan and swallowing techniques and providing emotional support to patient and significant other are key nursing interventions.

The nurse should assess the patient's pain level prior to meals. If the patient has increased pain due to swallowing, administer analgesics 30 minutes before mealtime. Adequate analgesia is key to ensure the patient's comfort and helps to improve dietary intake.

Discharge Planning

The average length of stay (LOS) for an uncomplicated tracheostomy is 3 to 5 days. A plan of care must begin prior to the patient's admission to ensure both a timely and safe discharge home. Evaluation of the patient and significant other's ability and readiness to learn and care for the tracheostomy should be assessed early and continue throughout the hospitalization. An introduction to the surgical procedure, the tracheostomy tube, and teaching booklets on tracheostomy care should be given to patients prior to their admission. This prepares the patient and significant other for surgery and the subsequent discharge home.

Home care can be challenging for patients with limitations in vision, mental status, mobility, and manual dexterity.[13] Extra time needs to be given to these patients to meet the goal of a safe and timely discharge. In some situations, a patient may not be able to return home after hospitalization due to the inability of the patient or caregiver to demonstrate safe care. If a potential for placement following hospitalization is identified, the process should be started early as there is often a waiting list for admission to facilities that may result in an increase in the hospital LOS.

Patients capable of self-care should begin to provide their own care as early as possible. Patients should not be sent home until they and/or their caregiver can independently demonstrate proper care of the tracheostomy. Tracheostomy care includes: cleaning the inner cannula, suctioning the tracheostomy tube, changing tracheostomy ties or holder, changing the tracheostomy tube, use of supplemental humidification or oxygen, and care of the stoma. Additionally, the patient and significant other need to be able to use alternative communication techniques; provide incision and skin care; and manage nutritional needs. The home health nurse can assist with changing of the tracheostomy tube ties, tube changes, and reinforce the education. The home health nurse's goal is to ensure the patient and significant other can provide all care independently. The home health nurse will continue to teach at home until this goal is met.

Equipment needs for care of a tracheostomy at home include the following: an extra tracheostomy tube, suction catheters, suction machine, sterile water and normal saline solution, compressor for humidification, tracheostomy masks and tubing, tracheostomy care kits to clean reusable inner cannulas or extra disposable inner cannulas, gloves, tracheostomy ties or holder, hydrogen peroxide, cotton swabs, stoma covers, tracheostomy dressings, normal saline for instillation into the tracheostomy, and teaching materials. Much of the equipment used in the home will be different from the hospital equipment. Arrangements should be made prior to discharge for delivery of equipment so that the patient has everything needed upon arrival to the home. The medical supplier will review how to operate the humidifier and suction machine with the patient upon arrival home or in advance with the caregiver. Planning is imperative to coordinate equipment delivery and instruction.

Financial planning including a review of insurance coverage for home care needs to be investigated early in the patient's hospitalization. If the patient has no insurance coverage for home care, it is vital to ensure that the patient or caregiver can provide care independently prior to discharge. The professional nurse and social worker can investigate foundations or charitable agencies for funding and support to help meet home care needs.

If the care required is complicated or if the home health care agency is not familiar with tracheostomy care the nurse should provide detailed written instructions and an offer for the home health nurse to observe the required care at the time of the referral. Multimedia instructions including written materials and video and/or audiotapes should be provided to the patient, significant others, and home health agency.

The nurse should review changes in activities of daily living (ADLs) and adaptations the patient needs to make with the patient and significant others. Precautions need to be taken when the patient showers or bathes; the patient is instructed to avoid the introduction of water into the stoma. A commercial shower shield can be purchased or a baby bib with the plastic side outward to repel the water can be worn. The tracheostomy opening may be camouflaged with commercial coverings such as scarves, neckties, jewelry, or gauze without compromising the airway. In addition to the aesthetic properties, a protective covering will help prevent foreign bodies and cold air from entering the tra-

chea. A moist covering or bib also can be used to add moisture to the air breathed.

Normal sexual activity can be resumed as soon as the patient and significant other are ready; however, the disfigurement related to tracheostomy placement will likely alter a patient's self-image. Body image issues often confront the patient and significant other once they leave the supportive and sheltered hospital environment. The patient and significant other may benefit from counseling. The social worker should begin working with the patient and significant other in the hospital as well as facilitate connecting them with organizations or support groups following discharge or professional mental health therapists if needed. The patient and significant other should be provided with information and referral numbers to agencies available in their area for continued emotional support such as the American Cancer Society (ACS). The social worker can also provide guidance to those patients with concerns regarding the ability to return to work following discharge and provide assistance in understanding the many processes to ensure continued employment or disability if needed. This may help minimize loss of income.

The social worker and nurse should address any substance abuse such as addiction to tobacco, drugs, or alcohol during hospitalization to increase the patient's chances for a healthier and safer lifestyle. Appropriate referrals to local agencies and organizations should be given to the patient prior to discharge. The patient and significant other should also be made aware that social services are available at home via the home health agency.

The home health nurse should monitor and report psychosocial problems, such as anxiety, depression, or difficulty coping with the illness once the patient is home. Home counseling may be available through the home health agency for psychological support to homebound patients. This information should also be available in the physician's office during follow-up visits.

The patient and significant other should be provided with resources for support and emergency care. With the patient's permission, the nurse should inform the patient's local emergency response department for the completely voiceless patient living alone. The emergency response team should be made aware that should a call come from this patient's address that they have a tracheostomy who cannot verbally communicate. An emergency identification bracelet or tag stating that the patient is a neck-breather is necessary to alert any emergency team that may be called upon to provide care to this patient. Techniques of mouth-to-tracheostomy (or stoma for the total laryngectomy) or bag-to-stoma resuscitation should be discussed with the significant other for use during a potential respiratory arrest.

In conclusion, caring for a patient with a tracheostomy will require a multidisciplinary team to provide a safe hospitalization stay and discharge. The nurse will work collaboratively with colleagues that include physicians, a speech and swallow therapist, dietician, physical and occupational therapists, respiratory therapists, social worker, behavioral medicine professionals, case managers, insurance carriers, home health professionals, medical equipment supplier, rehabilitation facilities, and long-term care facilities. All consultations and discussions regarding the patient's plan of care and discharge should be started as early as possible and reviewed daily with the entire multidisciplinary team and patient during hospitalization to facilitate returning the patient home in a safe and timely manner.

REFERENCES

1. Sigler BA, Schuring LT. *Ear, Nose, and Throat Disorders: A Clinical Nursing Series.* St. Louis, Mo: Mosby-Yearbook; 1993:250.
2. Conlan A, Kopec SE, Silva WE. Tracheostomy. In: Irwin, RS, Rippe JM, eds. *Irwin and Rippe's Intensive Care Medicine.* 5th ed. Philadelphia, Pa: Lippincott Williams & Wilkins; 2003:150–160.
3. Roman M. Tracheostomy tubes. *Medsurg Nursing.* 2005;14(2);143–145.
4. Hickey MM. Focus on tracheostomy, *Perspectives,* 2003;4(3):1–8.
5. Decker GM. Myers J. Commonly used herbs: implications for clinical practice. *Clin J Oncol Nurs.* 2001;5(2):insert 1–11.
6. Dawson CJ. Patient assessment. In: Clarke LK, Dropkin MJ, eds. *Head and Neck Cancer.* Pittsburgh, Pa: Oncology Nursing Press; 2006:35–48.
7. Hess DR. Tracheostomy tubes and related appliances. *Resp Care.* 2005; 50(4);497–510.
8. Hudak M, Bond-Domb A. Postoperative head and neck cancer patients with artificial airways: the effect of saline lavage on tracheal mucus evacuation and oxygen saturation. *ORL-Head Neck Nurs.* 1996;14:17–21.
9. Seay SJ, Gay SL, Strauss M. Tracheostomy emergencies: correcting accidental decannulation or displaced tracheotomy tube. *Am J Nurs.* 2002;102(3):59–63.
10. Bourjeily G, Habr F, Supinski G. Review of tracheostomy usage: complications and decannulation procedures. Part II. *Clin Pulm Med.* 2002;9(5):273–278.
11. Happ MB, Roesch T, Kagan SH. Communication needs, methods, and perceived

voice quality following head and neck surgery: a literature review. *Cancer Nurs.* 2004;27(1):1-9.

12. Higgins DM, Maclean JT. Dysphagia in the patient with tracheostomy: six cases of inappropriate cuff deflation or removal. *Heart Lung.* 1997;26(3):215-220.

13. Mainarich K, Silverstein P. Is your patient ready for home health care? *Nursing.* 2005;35(12):32hn6-32hn7.

CHAPTER 10

Long-Term Care of Patients with a Tracheostomy

DAVID A. NACE
ANDREA R. FOX

RATIONALE FOR UNDERSTANDING LONG-TERM CARE OPTIONS

There have been a number of dramatic changes in the field of health care over the past several decades. One of the most important of these has been the trend to shorten hospital lengths of stay in an effort to curtail rising health-care costs and reduce the incidence of iatrogenic complications. According to the Centers for Disease Control and Prevention, average hospital lengths of stay have been declining since 1970.[1] In the year 2000, the overall average length of stay for all diagnoses was approximately 5.9 days. Concurrent with the reduction in length of stay is a shift toward increased usage of formal home and long-term care services. In fact, between 1985 and 1999, overall hospital discharges to long-term care sites doubled.[2]

Given these changes in health care utilization, it should come as no surprise that the demographics of tracheostomy patients is evolving as well. The number of tracheotomies has risen over time, and data suggest this increase is substantial.[3] For example, a recent analysis of all patients undergoing tracheostomy for prolonged mechanical ventilation in North Carolina between 1993 and 2002 demonstrated a 200% increase over the decade.[4] Interestingly, this increase was disproportionate to the smaller rise in incidence of prolonged mechanical ventilation suggesting additional factors are important in determining tracheostomy rates. In part, improvements in short-term outcomes may be driving the increase in tracheostomy placement. Although current evidence does not firmly support a reduction in short-term mortality or pneumonia rates, duration of mechanical ventilation and length of critical care unit stays appear to be shortened.[5] Increased hospital reimbursement rates also have been implicated as an important factor in the increased placement of tracheotomies.[3] However, other variables important in the decision of if and when to place a tracheostomy remain to be clarified.[6,7]

Whatever the cause in the rise in use of tracheostomy, patients are spending less time in acute care settings and more are being discharged to postacute care settings. For instance, in the North Carolina study mentioned above, there was a reduction of in-hospital mortality (39 to 25%) and median length of stay (47 to 33 days). Interestingly, though, the proportion of patients being able to be discharged home independently decreased from 26 to 9% and the admissions to long-term care or rehab facilities doubled from 28 to 58%. Other studies support the risk of increased functional dependency as well as significant postacute care mortality and significant readmission rates. These findings are particularly noticeable for the elderly.[8-10]

Two important management issues arise as a result of increased dependency. First, most patients being discharged will need skilled care services provided by nursing facilities, rehabilitation facilities, or certified home care agencies. Whenever a patient moves from one health care setting to another, she or he is at risk for inadvertent complications in care. Consistent with the American Geriatric Society's position statement, *Improving*

the Quality of Transitional Care for Persons with Complex Care Needs, clinicians caring for tracheostomy patients must be knowledgeable about the various postacute care settings.[11] They must also be actively involved in the discharge planning process. Second, it is important to carefully involve patients and families early in the decision-making process when tracheostomy is being considered, as it is readily apparent that most patients will require extended care following their acute stay and be at increased risk of adverse outcomes.

WHAT IS A LONG-TERM CARE FACILITY?

Although the term *long-term care* is most often associated with nursing facilities or nursing homes, long-term care should be thought of as a spectrum of services. Included in this spectrum are assisted living programs, subacute or transitional units, chronic disease hospitals, respite care services, nursing facilities, and long-term acute care hospitals (LTACH).[12,13] The focus and care provided in each of these settings varies. Table 10–1 briefly describes these service sites. Generally, the most appropriate *institutional* site for a patient being discharged with a new tracheostomy would be either a nursing facility, a subacute unit, or LTACH. These facilities provide skilled services throughout the day, matching the increased care needs of tracheostomy patients. As assisted living or personal care centers provide relatively limited services, which generally do not include round the clock skilled nursing, they are not an ideal setting for the patient with a new tracheotomy.

Table 10–1. Types of Institutional Long-Term Care Settings

Site	Other Names Used	Description of Care Provided
Assisted Living	Personal care Boarding home care	Residents are provided room and board. Some assistance is required with instrumental activities of daily living such as housework, bathing, meal preparation, and administering medication. Skilled nursing services are not available, and in general, the residents are not fully dependent on others for care. On-site physician visits are not required.
Nursing Facility	Nursing home, *skilled nursing,* and *intermediate care* are older terms that are occasionally used to separate nursing facility care into more and less extensive service requirements, depending on the need for skilled nursing care such as frequent dressing changes, intravenous medications and fluids, and so on.	Residents require a great deal of assistance with simple daily activities such as toileting, bathing, dressing, and eating. Skilled services, including education, may be provided. Physical and occupational therapy may also be provided. Onsite physician visits must occur every 30 to 60 days.
Subacute Unit	Transitional care unit	A nursing facility that provides skilled nursing or rehabilitative care to residents for short durations before they return home or are placed in a nursing facility. On-site physician visits must occur every 30 days, but many facilities require weekly or more frequent physician visits.
Long-Term Acute Care Hospitals	LTAC or LTACH units	These are facilities licensed as acute care hospitals, but are designed for high acuity, technology-dependent patients requiring prolonged care stays. On-site physician visits occur daily.

continues

Table 10–1. *continued*

Site	Other Names Used	Description of Care Provided
Respite Care Services		Services that may be provided in a variety of care levels, such as assisted living or nursing facilities. The level of care would depend upon the need of the patient. Use of respite care services is meant to provide relief to a caregiver for an extended period of time for personal leave or emergencies. Generally these services are short-term, that is less than 3 months.
		Physician visits would depend upon the site in which care is provided as listed above.

An example of why clinicians must recognize differences among care settings occurs whenever a patient who has been residing at an assisted living center is admitted to the hospital, and undergoes a tracheostomy. Following the tracheostomy, the patient's postacute care needs will usually exceed the capabilities of the assisted living facility. In such cases, at least temporary placement in a nursing facility or LTACH would be more appropriate. The hospital social worker or case manager is often familiar with local or regional facilities and can be an invaluable resource to clinicians and patients when deciding about discharge plans.

Nursing Facilities, Subacute Facilities, and Transitional Care Units

Currently there are approximately 16,000 nursing facilities in the United States, providing care to an estimated 1.5 mil-lion nursing facility residents.[14] Despite the differences in terminology, *nursing homes, subacute units*, and *transitional care units* are all variants of the nursing home. The major difference between them is the degree of focus on rehabilitation or specialty care as well as the length of stay. Subacute facilities and transitional care units tend to provide short-term care as opposed to nursing facilities where indefinite stays are possible. As noted in the introduction to this chapter, nursing facilities now represent the largest hospital discharge destination of patients undergoing tracheostomy.[4]

The prevalence of tracheostomy patients will vary by facility. Overall, based on Online Survey, Certification, and Reporting System (OSCAR) data from the Centers for Medicare and Medicaid Services, approximately 1% of residents in nursing facilities have a tracheostomy.[15] This means that many facilities care for only an occasional resident with a tracheostomy. However, there is widespread variability among facilities. Some nursing facilities, such as subacute units, may specialize in caring for this population and thus have a higher percentage of patients who have a tracheotomy.

This is not to say that nursing facilities with a low prevalence of tracheotomies should not provide care to these patients. As subacute facilities, transitional care units, and LTACH generally provide short stays only, patients or their families will either gain the skills necessary to care for the tracheostomy at home, or the patient will be transferred to another nursing facility for extended custodial care. Thus, it is important for nursing facilities to develop a comprehensive approach to tracheostomy care. A comprehensive plan should address regular education of staff as well as frequent reviewing and updating of tracheostomy care policies and procedures. Preferably sites for discharge should be selected on the existence of such plans. Sample policies and procedures are included in Appendix 10-A at the end of this chapter.

There are some unique features of nursing facilities that may influence the clinician when deciding on a postacute site of care. First, there is no requirement for daily physician visits in nursing homes. As nursing facilities are focused on skilled nursing care, physicians are only required to visit patients once every 30 or 60 days. This may influence decisions on site of care for patients who have more complex health care needs. Second, nursing homes often have high staff turnover rates. The average annual turnover rate for nurses in Pennsylvania nursing homes is around 50%.[15] Thus, considering the frequency of patients with a tracheotomy in nursing facilities, the nursing facility must make sure that the current staff has been adequately trained in tracheostomy care procedures.

Long-Term Acute Care Hospitals

The LTACH is a relatively new postacute option for care in the past decade. The LTACH is an acute care hospital that accepts patients requiring prolonged lengths of stay and who are dependent on high-technology care. Such patients may even require ongoing intensive care unit (ICU) services.[12] Long-term acute care hospitals are exempt from the Medicare prospective payment system due to the average lengths of stay being greater than 25 days. The majority of patients being treated in LTACH require prolonged mechanical ventilation due to acute medical illnesses and tracheostomy is commonly found among this population of patients.[8] The LTACH is not designed to be a rehabilitation facility, but rather is meant to provide temporary care to a highly specific group of critically ill patients.[16] Still, education of the patient and family regarding tracheostomy care should be part of the patient's care plan.

GENERAL ISSUES FOR INSTITUTIONAL PATIENTS

Reasons for Placement

The reasons for postacute placement following tracheostomy have not been well studied but most likely relate to several factors. Caregiver issues are suspected of playing a major role. The simple lack of having any caregiver at home, or lack of a capable caregiver, presents an obvious barrier to a person trying to return home following tracheostomy. This is particularly true for older and more dependent patients where family members usually serve this role of caregiver. Whereas home health agencies can be used, their services are mostly limited to a few visits per week and should augment another caregiver's role. Although it is possible for a patient to privately hire paid caregivers, cost and accessibility are significant barriers. For patients who have a willing and capable caregiver at home, the issue of caregiver depression and burnout are substantial concerns. In fact, there is evidence that caregivers of patients who have a tracheostomy may have higher depression scores compared to other caregiver groups.[17,18] Age appears to be related to postacute placement with studies showing elderly patients being more likely to die or be discharged to long-term care facilities.[3,4]

Such a link is consistent with the authors' review of administrative data of patients undergoing tracheostomy at the University of Pittsburgh Medical Center from 1995 to 1997. In this review, patients discharged to a nursing home after tracheostomy were significantly older than those discharged home. The mean age for those discharged home was 53 years, compared with 62 years for those admitted to a long-term care facility. When patients having a diagnosis of cancer were analyzed separately, the age difference was even more marked. Although this information is limited, we postulate this reflects greater comorbidity and lessened social support among older adults undergoing tracheostomy (unpublished data). Cognitive impairment and anticipated decline in functional status, as expected in patients with cancer or severe lung disease, are also likely contributors. There are little or no published data formally linking cognition or functional status with long-term care placement of tracheostomy patients, although baseline functional status is linked to 1-year mortality in LTCAH patients.

Care Policies

Well-written tracheostomy care policies and procedures are essential in long-term care facilities, especially for facilities having low prevalence rates of such patients. Good tracheostomy policies and procedures serve several important functions. These include providing the rationale for a given procedure, giving concise instructions to carry out the task, and defining who is responsible for each part of the process. Well-written policies and procedures also ultimately allow for the development of quality improvement monitors. These monitors are a means for determining the adequacy and appropriateness of the care delivered to the patient with a tracheostomy. If quality improvement monitors uncover problems or noncompliance with policies, process revision and education can then be instituted to improve care. Of note, although the federal regulations governing nursing facilities are quite extensive and do mention tracheostomy care, their attention to tracheostomy care is extremely limited.[19] The content of these regulations does not help to establish thorough facility plans for tracheostomy care. Facility staff should seek outside input on tracheostomy care if they are uncomfortable with their knowledge base.

Attention to care policies and process are important from a regulatory and legal perspective as well. The current federal long-term care survey process targets all tracheostomy patients for in-depth review of care. There are case examples in which facilities have failed to follow their care policies leading to patient harm and regulatory citation.[20,21] Policies pertinent to patients who have a tracheostomy should include those addressing the cleaning of the cannulas, the process to follow in the event of accidental decannulation, as well as how changes in patient condition are reported to physicians, how physicians are expected to respond, and how patient rights and dignity are maintained.

Care Plans

Besides having updated policies, another critical component is developing a personalized care plan. Federal nursing home licensure regulations require nursing facilities to have individualized care plans that address conditions a patient faces.[19] Individual goals for the resident having a tracheostomy should be established based on the circumstances. For instance, teaching self-care may not be important for the resident who is admitted for terminal care or the resident with advanced cognitive impairment. Learning self-care would be appropriate if the resident were to return home or even if he or she were planning on staying in the facility and is physically and cognitively capable of doing so. In the latter case, promoting independence in self-care would be important in maximizing a person's physical and emotional functioning.

Interdisciplinary Care

A team approach is necessary for managing the patient with a tracheostomy in the long-term care setting. Such patients have diverse nursing, rehabilitative, medical, and psychosocial needs. Skilled nursing staff is generally responsible for the actual care and cleaning of the tracheostomy. Some facilities tend to limit the number of nurses providing skilled tracheostomy care; however, all nursing staff should be educated on the signs and symptoms of infections and other common problems. Also, all nursing staff should be familiar with the management of common emergencies such as accidental decannulation. We have noted a case in which a facility had failed to broadly cross-train staff on emergency care, resulting in a facility citation for inadequate care.[20] Facility leadership should remember that emergencies can happen at any point, and thus their staff must be broadly prepared for the common situations.

Other disciplines crucial to the care of patients with a tracheostomy in the long-term care setting include speech-language-pathologists (SLP), nutritionists, respiratory care therapists, pastoral care specialists, social services, as well as the patient's family or home caregivers. The SLP is responsible for developing and improving speech and other communication skills. In addition, she or he can help with other common comorbid problems such as dysphagia, cognitive impairment, and hearing problems. Nutritionists can help assess for appropriate dietary orders, addressing caloric intake and specific nutritional needs. Unlike hospitals and LTACH, most nursing facilities do not have respiratory care therapists on staff. Medicare reimbursement for respiratory services is limited to the short-term Part A services only, typically lasting from a few days to no more than 100 days. However, for nursing facilities caring for patients with a tracheostomy, it is possible to contract for these services through outside organizations if a patient has special needs or if the facility feels they can not meet some specialized needs. Under such agreements, some facilities can work with the contracted respiratory therapists to better train their staff, augmenting the services they provide to their other residents. Although one would assume that having a respiratory therapist present in a nursing facility would increase the quality of general pulmonary care provided to all residents, adequate studies have not been done to support this argument. Pastoral care can help residents, including those without religious affiliations, deal with their illness from a spiritual sense. This is important given the limited prognosis of many tracheostomy patients living in the long-term care setting. Likewise, an involved social worker is necessary to assist families with caregiver stress and conflicts as well as with assistance in the discharge process for those patients returning home.

Attending Physicians

Each patient admitted to a nursing facility or a LTACH must be under the care of an attending physician. This may or may not be a physician with whom the patient is familiar. Regardless, the attending physician must actively participate in the care and discharge planning process. Although regulations stipulate a minimum visit frequency of every 30 or 60 days for nursing facilities, patients with a tracheostomy have complex needs and thus more frequent visits may be required. Under updated CMS guidelines, visits that are medical necessary can be made more frequently, up to daily, in the nursing facility setting. In the LTACH setting, daily physician visits are required.

Responsibilities of the attending physician include: the ongoing management of acute and chronic medical problems; the routine assessment for causes of delay in rehabilitation progress such as complications due to depression, delirium, or medication side effects; ensuring responsive coverage when she or he is away;

and the timely signing of orders and other documents such as physical, occupational, and speech therapy certification forms. The attending physician must also be responsive to patient and family inquiries and should actively participate in appropriate advance care planning. To meet these responsibilities, the attending physician must be familiar and comfortable interacting with the different team members caring for the patient, addressing concerns raised by others, and ensuring that the care being provided is based on sound medical principles. These responsibilities are consistent with the recommendations of the American Geriatric Society on improving transitional care in persons with complex care needs.[11]

For many patients with a tracheostomy, outside follow-up and consultation with an otolaryngologist, or pulmonary specialist is recommended. To ensure continuity, the specialist chosen would ideally be the person who has taken care of the resident previously. It should be emphasized that, although a resident may have follow-up care arranged with a specialist, direct communication between that specialist, the attending physician, and/or the nursing facility team must occur. Any specialist following a resident of a nursing facility should be willing and available to provide a timely response to questions concerning the residents.

Medical Director

The medical director is a very important team member. Federal regulations for nursing facilities establish the role of the medical director as coordinating the medical care of the facility and implementing policies of resident care. The regulations specify that the medical director must do more than approve policies.[19] The medical director must be involved in the development, implementation, and assessment of the policies. Many medical directors in the past have spent little time focusing on these duties. However, the increasing complexity of long-term care patients as well as recent changes to the federal interpretive guidelines have placed greater emphasis on the role of the medical director.[22] The medical director should participate in establishing and evaluating policies for tracheostomy care as described above.

To summarize the approach to tracheostomy care in institutional long-term care settings, policies need to be established, monitored, and revised as needed. An interdisciplinary team, that includes the attending physician and medical director, needs to coordinate efforts in providing care. Effective communication between team members must occur. Education is crucial for all team members including the resident and his or her family as they form the central focus of the team's activities.

HOME CARE

Certified Home Health Services

As noted in the introduction of this chapter, the patient and family must be included early in discussions regarding tracheostomy placement. Although the utilization of institutional long-term care services following the acute placement of a tracheostomy is increasing, especially for older patients, a smaller number of patients may still be able to return directly home. Such patients will need to be motivated, have adequate cognitive

and emotional abilities to handle the tracheostomy, and should have access to caregivers who are adequately trained. Given the decrease in hospital lengths of stay, there is increasing difficulty in providing much of the patient and family education necessary to prepare for tracheostomy care in the home setting. Thus, there is an appropriate role for use of certified home health agencies. Medicare certified home health agencies provide skilled nursing services for time-limited periods in the patient's home. Patients must have a skilled nursing need, have services ordered by a physician, and the patient must be confined to the home. Unfortunately, the definition of homebound has been misunderstood.[23] According to the Medicare definition, this does not mean that patients are unable to leave their homes, but rather that absences from the home are for health care treatments, or if they are nonmedically related, occur infrequently or for short durations.[24,25]

There are several roles that home health services can provide. Obviously home health agencies can provide direct care of the tracheostomy. However, as home health services cannot be continued indefinitely, patients with a tracheostomy or their caregivers must assume some of the care responsibilities. Thus, home health staff should educate patients and their caregivers on how to care for the tracheostomy, how to monitor the site, and how to respond to common care situations such as emergencies. Home health agencies also can be used to reassess patient or caregiver skills and compliance if there is a concern that care techniques have declined. In addition, they can help ensure a safe and clean environment of the patient with a tracheostomy in the home.

Caregiver Education

Education of the patient and caregiver is critical to the successful home transition of tracheostomy patients.[26] Adequate knowledge of and ability in the day to day management of the tracheostomy, as well as the knowledge and management of complications is essential. The patient and caregivers must participate actively in performing the care while being closely observed and provided with useful, nonthreatening feedback. He or she should be encouraged to ask questions during the training process. Proficiency and comfort come with the extent of education and quality of experience given. Patients and their caregivers also need to be aware of the indications for the tracheostomy, the short- and long-term goals of care, and general health issues. There is also a need to define how to communicate with the health care team that cares for the patient including any home health agency nurses, aides, or therapists; the physician overseeing home health services; and pertinent specialists involved in the patient's care.

Having a comprehensive, easy to understand, home care manual will help in this process. Several manuals are available and caregivers find these very helpful. The caregiver can refer to and review the information as necessary. Kingston and coworkers have described their experience in the development of a home care manual for pediatric patients.[27] This study reported on the efforts to develop a manual and evaluate the understanding and usefulness of its content to parents. Parents found the manual very useful in providing specific information needed to provide care to their children at home. All the parents surveyed felt that such a home care manual should be provided at the time of discharge.[28]

Home care manuals should include background information on tracheostomy, procedures for caring for the tracheostomy, and information on what to do in an emergency. The manual should be easy to read, provide useful photographs and figures, and should be updated from time to time as necessary. It is also helpful to include written personalized information for the patient if the procedure to be followed deviates in any way from what is presented in the manual (eg, if the changes of cannula are to be more or less frequent, etc).

Physician Involvement with Home Health Services

Whereas home health care services must be ordered by a physician, direct physician care in the home setting is not included as a routine part of these services. Under the home health service benefit, the physician's role is that of coordination and oversight. This means that a patient must have a physician identified who is available to communicate with the home health agency staff, address relevant condition changes, sign verbal orders to the home care nurse, and provide written certification of the continuing need for skilled home nursing services. The amount of time spent in these activities can be significant for patients with a tracheostomy given their complex needs. In the past, reimbursement mechanisms did not exist to compensate physicians for the time spent in such communication and certification activities. Thus, many physicians were reluctant participants. However, Medicare has added several mechanisms to overcome barriers to home health service oversight and coordination activities. In 1995, Medicare began paying for care plan oversight in the home setting.[29] Care plan oversight provides reimbursement for the physician supervision of complex, multidisciplinary home health agency services necessitating regular physician input into care plans, review of subsequent patient status reports, review of laboratory and other studies, communication with other health care professionals involved in the patient's care, and adjustment of medical therapy. The services are time based and must involve 30 minutes or more each calendar month. Physicians must document the time spent in care plan oversight activities, and use the appropriate Current Procedural Terminology (CPT code G0181). Subsequently, in January 2000, Medicare authorized a separate payment for signing home health certification forms as well as for review of the patient's assessment by the home care agency, notation of response to treatment, ongoing communication with the home care agency, and assurance of continuing need for the home care agency's services. Home health certification and recertification services are submitted using the CPT codes G0180 and G0179, respectively. The development of these codes is a major step forward for physicians managing complex patients with a tracheostomy in the home care setting. Physicians should review their carrier's instructions and documentation requirements on the use of these codes.[23,30,31]

Caregiver Support

Caregiver burden and stress are well-recognized problems among family members of chronically ill patients.[32,33] In general, caregivers are at an increased risk for depression, burnout, and poor personal health. The same appears to be true for caregivers of patients receiving long-term ventilatory support. A study looking at caregiver outcomes after hospital discharge for patients receiving long-term ventilation showed increased burden, depression, and poorer physical health 6 months after hospital discharge.[17] Because of the prevalence of adverse outcomes, caregivers of tracheostomy patients should be screened by the treatment team for depression, burnout, and health status. If concern arises, interventions such as respite care, increased home support, or placement can be arranged to alleviate the burden and, one hopes, lessen the impact on the caregiver and patient.

Communication

One potential pitfall to avoid is the all too frequent problem of lack of communication among team members about the patient's status, care goals, and current levels of service. In the home care setting, the authors have witnessed situations in which multiple home services were involved and there was poor communication among them. In such cases, care provided may be duplicative or even medically unnecessary. Having one attending physician who oversees the home services is very important. If other physicians or health professionals are involved in the care and wish to make changes in the treatment regimen, they should only do so after consulting with the primary attending physician.

REFERENCES

1. Centers for Disease Control and Prevention. *Trends in Health and Aging*. Retrieved December 6, 2006; from http://www.cdc.gov/nchs/agingact.htm

2. Bernstein A, Hing E, Moss A, et al. *Health Care in America: Trends in Utilization.* Hyattsville, Md: National Center for Health Statistics; 2003.

3. Dewar D, Kurek C, Lambrinos J, et al. Patterns for costs and outcomes for patients with prolonged mechanical ventilation undergoing tracheostomy: an analysis of discharges under diagnosis-related group 483 in New York State from 1992-1996. *Critical Care Med.* 1999;27(12):2640-2647.

4. Cox C, Carson S, Holmes G, et al. Increase in tracheostomy for prolonged mechanical ventilation in North Carolina, 1993-2002. *Critical Care Med.* 2004; 32(11):2219-2226.

5. Griffiths J, Barber V, Morgan L, et al. Systematic review and meta-analysis of studies of the timing of tracheostomy in adult patients undergoing artificial ventilation. *Br Med J.* 2005;330:1243-1247.

6. Heffner J. Timing of tracheostomy in mechanically ventilated patients. *Am Rev Resp Dis.* 1993;147:768-771.

7. Maziak D, Meade M, Todd T. The timing of tracheostomy: a systematic review. *Chest.* 1998;114(2):605-609.

8. Carson S, Bach P, Brzozowski L, et al. Outcomes after long-term acute care. *Am J Resp Crit Care Med.* 1999;159: 1568-1573.

9. Douglas S, Daly B, Gordon N, et al. Survival and quality of life: short-term versus long-term ventilator patients. *Crit Care Med.* 2002;30(12):2655-2662.

10. Nasraway S, Button G, Rand W, et al. Survivors of catastrophic illness: outcome after direct transfer from intensive care to extended care facilities. *Crit Care Med.* January 2000;28(1):19-25.

11. Coleman E, Boult C. Improving the quality of transitional care for persons with complex care needs. *J Am Geriatr Soc.* 2003;51(4):556-557.

12. Hill-Lamb M. More alphabet soup: LTAC. How does long-term acute care fit into the health care continuum? *Surg Serv Manag.* 1995;1(3):31-35.

13. Levenson S. The spectrum of long term care sites, programs, and services. In: Levenson S, ed. *Medical Direction in Long Term Care: A Guidebook for the Future.* Durham, NC: Academic Press; 1993.

14. Ouslander J, Osterweil D, Morley J. Demographics and economics of nursing home care. In: Ouslander J, Osterweil D, Morley J, eds. *Medical Care in the Nursing Home.* 2nd ed. New York, NY: McGraw-Hill; 1997.

15. Decker F, Gruhn P, Matthews-Martin L, et al. *Results of the 2002 AHCA Survey of Nursing Staff Vacancy and Turnover in Nursing Homes.* Retrieved July 7, 2006 from http://www.ahca.org/research/rpt_vts2002_final.pdf

16. Murer C. The LTCACH in rehab clothing. *Rehab Management.* 2005:44-46.

17. Douglas S, Daly B. Caregivers of long-term ventilator patients: physical and psychological outcomes. *Chest.* 2003; 123(4):1073-1081.

18. Ferrario S, Zotti A, Zaccaria S, et al. Caregiver strain associated with tracheostomy in chronic respiratory failure. *Chest.* 2001;119(5):1498-1502.

19. Centers for Medicare and Medicaid Services. State Operations Manual: Appendix PP—Guidance to Surveyors for Long Term Care Facilities. Retrieved December 6, 2006 from http://cms.hhs.gov/manuals/Downloads/som107ap_pp_guidelines_ltcf.pdf

20. State of Florida DOAH. Agency for Health Care Administration, Petitioner, v. Perry Healthcare Associates, LLC, d/b/a Marshall Health and Rehabilitation Center, Respondent. Case No. 04-1198. http://www.doah.state.fl.us/ros/2004/04-1198.doc. June 13, 2005.

21. Tammelleo A. Nurses refuse to follow orders: catastrophic results. Case on point. Szczuvelek v. Harborside Healthcare Woods Edge. *Nursing Law's Regan Report.* 2005;45(9):2.

22. *American Medical Directors Association. Roles and Responsibilities of the*

Medical Director in the Nursing Home. Retrieved December 6, 2003 from http:// www.amda.com/governance/resolu tions/a06.cfm.

23. Moore K. An update on certifying home health care. *Fam Prac Manag.* 2001;8:16.
24. Centers for Medicare and Medicaid Services. Medicare Benefit Policy Manual. Chapter 15—*Covered Medical and Other Health Services.* Retrieved December 6, 2006; from http://www.cms.hhs. gov/manuals/Downloads/bp102c15.pdf
25. Centers for Medicare and Medicaid Services. Medicare Benefit Policy Manual: Chapter 7—Home Health Services. Retrieved December 6, 2006; from http:// www.cms.hhs.gov/manuals/Downloads/ bp102c07.pdf
26. Fiske E. Effective strategies to prepare infants and families for home tracheostomy care [Advertisement]. *Neonat Care.* 2004;4(1):42-53.
27. Kingston L, Brodsky L, Volk M, et al. Development and assessment of a home care tracheostomy manual. *Int J Pediatr Otorhinolaryngol.* 1995;32:213-222.
28. Johnson J, Wagner R, Sigler B. Disposable inner cannula tracheostomy tube: a prospective clinical trial. *Otolaryngol Head Neck Surg.* 1988;99:83-84.
29. Centers for Medicare and Medicaid Services. Medicare Claims Processing Manual: Chapter 12—Physician/Nonphysician Practitioners. Retrieved December 6, 2006; from http://www.cms.hhs.gov/ manuals/downloads/clm104c12.pdf
30. Baker B. *Medicare Changes Some Rules on Home Health Billing.* Accessed November 28, 2006, from http://www. acponline.org/journals/news/mar01/ homebilling.htm
31. Hughes C. Coding and documentation. *Fam Pract Manag.* 2006;13:30.
32. Covinsky K, Goldman L, Cook E F, et al. The impact of serious illness on patients' families. SUPPORT Investigators. Study to understand prognoses and preferences for outcomes and risks of treatment. *JAMA.* 1994;272(23):1839-1844.
33. Moore M, Zhu C, Clipp E. Informal costs of dementia care: estimates from the National Longitudinal Caregiver Study. *J Gerontol. Ser B, Psycholog Sci Soc Sci.* 2001;56:S219-S228.

APPENDIX 10-A

Care Policies and Procedures

CHANGING OR CLEANING THE INNER CANNULA

The inner cannula must be changed or cleaned regularly to ensure a patent airway. Inner cannulas may be either disposable or reusable. Disposable inner cannulas are discarded at each change and never reused. They offer ease of use, and as the cleaning step is eliminated, provide a time savings.[28] Their drawback is that they are relatively expensive. Their use is reasonable whenever competence in cleaning is suspect or when the changes must be made frequently. Reusable inner cannulas require thorough cleaning but may be more economical. Physicians, licensed nurses, or respiratory therapists may all perform inner cannula care. The frequency of cleaning/changing will vary and should be clarified with the treating physician. As a general reference in long-term care facilities, the usual frequency would be once each shift. However, whenever there is an indication that secretions have accumulated and may pose a threat to the airway, more frequent changes may be necessary. It is important to promptly notify the attending physician of any changes in the patient's condition.

POLICY TITLE: Tracheostomy Care Policy: Changing a Disposable Inner Cannula

POLICY STATEMENT

Tracheostomy care is performed a minimum of one time per shift using aseptic technique. It will be provided by a licensed nurse or a respiratory therapist, as appropriate.

PURPOSE

- To maintain patency of the airway;
- To keep the tracheostomy tube and surrounding area clean;
- To prevent excoriation of the skin around the tracheostomy tube.

PROCEDURE

1. Verify the need for changing the tube.
2. Clean the over-the-bed table.
3. Wash hands thoroughly.
4. Assemble the equipment and supplies, including a new disposable cannula, tracheostomy-care set, suction equipment and suction kit, sterile gloves, saline, sterile water, hydrogen peroxide, scissors, second tracheostomy set of same size.
5. The patient should be on her or his back, with the bed at a 45-degree angle, and should understand the planned procedure.
6. Provide privacy.
7. Initiate pulse oximetry monitoring.
8. Put on gloves and personal protection equipment as necessary, such as mask, gown.
9. Suction the patient as necessary.
10. Remove gloves and wash hands.
11. Open and prepare the tracheostomy care kit in a sterile fashion. Remember to put a sterile glove on one hand. Using this hand, separate the supplies onto a sterile field. Use

the ungloved hand to pour saline and peroxide onto the kit's solution trays or directly onto sterile 4×4 gauze sponges, depending on the contents of the kit. Using sterile procedures, put the remaining glove on the other hand.

12. Stabilize the neck plate of the tracheostomy with one hand and grasp the snap lock (Shiley tubes) with the other hand.
13. Squeeze the snap lock and pull the inner cannula from the outer cannula with an outward and downward motion.
14. Discard the old inner cannula.
15. Remove and discard the old tracheostomy dressing.
16. Clean the tracheostomy neck plate with the kit's cleaning sticks or 4×4 gauze sponges soaked with hydrogen peroxide. Dry with gauze sponge.
17. Clean around the stoma site using the cleaning sticks or sponges. Dry with gauze sponge.
18. Remove gloves, wash hands, and put on new gloves.
19. Pick up the new inner cannula and squeeze the snap-lock connector.
20. Place the new cannula into the outer cannula fully until it locks into place, remembering to hold the outer cannula steady.
21. Apply a clean dressing.

POLICY TITLE: Tracheostomy Care Policy: Cleaning a Reusable Inner Cannula

POLICY STATEMENT

Tracheostomy care is performed a minimum of one time per shift using aseptic technique. It will be provided by a licensed nurse or a respiratory therapist, as appropriate.

PURPOSE

▓ To maintain patency of the airway;
▓ To keep the tracheostomy tube and surrounding area clean;
▓ To prevent excoriation of the area around the tracheostomy tube.

PROCEDURE

1. Complete steps 1 through 11 as described above.
2. Stabilize the neck plate of the tracheostomy with one hand and twist counterclockwise to unlock (for Shiley tubes). Remove the inner cannula using an outward and downward motion.
3. Place the inner cannula into the hydrogen peroxide solution to soak.
4. If the inner cannula is metal, do not clean with hydrogen peroxide, use water only.
5. Clean around the stoma using applicator sticks or gauze sponges soaked in saline or hydrogen peroxide and dry.
6. Clean neck plate with peroxide and rinse with sterile water or saline using cotton applicators.
7. Clean inner cannula in the peroxide using tracheostomy brush or pipe cleaner.
8. After cleaning, rinse thoroughly with sterile water or saline and dry with 4×4 gauze.
9. Remove gloves, wash hands, and put on new gloves.
10. Place clean inner cannula into the outer cannula while holding neck plate stable.
11. Replace sponge under the neck plate.

OUTER CANNULA

The outer cannula is changed first in the hospital by the physician. Subsequent changes should be done on the advice of the physician and only after the caregiver has been adequately trained. There have been no randomized controlled trials to define the appropriate timing for changing the outer cannula. In long-term care facilities, a standard policy is to have the physician or respiratory therapist change the outer cannula every 1 to 3 months. More frequent changes may be needed depending on the presence of signs of infection or other problems. Because of the lack of data, the timing of and responsibility for changes are an important issues to be clarified with the otolaryngologist or pulmonary specialist.

One should remember to assess the patient constantly during the tube-changing process to ensure adequate airflow. Also, it is important to remember to have at least one spare tube of the same size on hand at all times. The obturator should also be saved and kept near the patient in a readily accessible location to aid in reinsertion of the tracheostomy tube.

POLICY TITLE: Procedure for changing the outer cannula (cuffless tube):

POLICY STATEMENT

Tracheostomy care is performed a minimum of one time per shift using aseptic technique. It will be provided by a licensed nurse or a respiratory therapist, as appropriate.

PURPOSE

- To maintain patency of the airway;
- To keep the tracheostomy tube and surrounding area clean;
- To prevent excoriation of the area around the tracheostomy tube.

PROCEDURE

1. Verify the need for changing the outer cannula.
2. Wash over-the-bed table.
3. Wash hands thoroughly.
4. Assemble the equipment and supplies, including a tracheostomy care kit, suction equipment and kit, sterile gloves, sterile gauze sponges, hydrogen peroxide, saline, sterile water, water soluble lubricant, scissors, and a second tracheostomy set with an obturator of the same size.
5. The patient should be on her or his back at a 45-degree angle and understand the planned procedure.
6. Provide privacy.
7. Initiate pulse oximetry monitoring.
8. Put on gloves and, if needed, personal protective equipment such as mask or gown.
9. Suction the patient as necessary.
10. Remove soiled sponges from around tracheostomy and discard.
11. Remove gloves, wash hands.
12. Prepare the tracheostomy ties as per usual procedure.
13. Open the new tracheostomy tube set and prepare tracheostomy care kit in usual sterile fashion. Remember to use sterile gloves.
14. Remove the inner cannula from the new tracheostomy tube. Insert the obturator into the new tube.

15. Attach the tracheostomy ties to the outer cannula.
16. Lubricate the end of the tracheostomy tube and obturator with a thin film of water-soluble lubricant.
17. Remove the old tracheostomy dressing and cut the ties holding the old tube in place with scissors.
18. Remove the entire old tube by grasping neck plate with the thumb and forefinger and pulling out and downward. Do not force when removing the tube.
19. Immediately insert the lubricated new tube and obturator with gentle pressure.
20. Hold the outer cannula in place and immediately remove the obturator.
21. Insert the inner cannula and lock it into place.
22. Still holding the outer cannula in place, secure the new tube with the tracheostomy ties. Make sure to allow one finger to fit beneath the ties.
23. Clean tracheostomy neck plate and stoma.
24. Apply a new tracheostomy dressing.

CHAPTER 11

Communication Options for Tracheostomy and Ventilator-Dependent Patients

MARTA S. KAZANDJIAN AND KAREN J. DIKEMAN

The ability to communicate with others is the essence of being human, maintaining connection to other people and exercising power over our environment.[1] Tracheostomy and ventilator dependence are associated with both serious and sometimes chronic illness, the loss of mobility, and—all too often—the loss of speech and communication. It is the role of the speech-language pathologist (SLP), in collaboration with other team members, to ensure that the patient with a tracheostomy who is ventilator-dependent has a consistent, reliable, and effective method of communication, whether oral/vocal or nonoral/nonvocal, throughout his or her hospitalization.

The speech-language pathologist usually takes the primary role in the management of communication impairment with this population but cannot do so effectively without the assistance of key members of the medical team. The term transdisciplinary has been used to describe one team format that is useful in dealing with this challenging population.[2] Transdisciplinary refers to a concept by which key team members share roles for the achievement of a particular treatment goal. For example, the speech-language pathologist and respiratory therapist are often the professionals who evaluate the tracheostomized patient for the use of a one-way tracheostomy speaking valve.

The speech-language pathologist has the expertise in management of the tracheostomy tube for purposes of communication and swallowing, but needs the assistance of professionals skilled in the care of the patient's airway during the evaluation and intervention process. Although scope of practice is maintained, boundaries may blur as team members strive to achieve their goals in the most effective manner.

The needs of these complex patients demand a carefully coordinated concept of care. Any policies and procedures designed to address management of the patient with a tracheostomy will incorporate appropriate team members and ensure that the role of each professional is delineated. Once the policy and procedures are developed, it will be clear which team members must receive special training in a particular area of care. For example, it is common in specialized tracheostomy and ventilator-dependent facilities, to credential speech-language pathologists and others in tracheal suctioning.[3]

TRACHEOSTOMY: IMPACT ON COMMUNICATION

Physiologic Impact: Redirection of Normal Airflow

Placement of a tracheostomy tube into the trachea interrupts the normal flow of air through the larynx. Because the tracheostomy tube is placed below the level of the larynx, most of the airflow, entering and leaving the airway through the path of least resistance, never reaches the vocal folds. This disturbance of normal airflow affects the entire respiratory-phonatory system. Loss of phonation and voice production is referred to as apho-

nia, whereas an impairment of voice production (such as a disturbance in quality or volume) is referred to as dysphonia.

Loss of Airflow to the Upper Airway

The size and type of tracheostomy tube usually determines whether any airflow will be diverted around the sides of the tracheostomy tube, possibly reaching the vocal folds. Many physicians use a sizing guideline that the tracheostomy tube should fill no more than two-thirds to three-quarters of the tracheal lumen.[4] However, adult tracheostomy tubes often fill most of the trachea. Although the larger size tracheostomy tube will lessen the resistance to inspired air, a larger tube will also block airflow to the vocal folds. Therefore, a patient may be aphonic because of the size of the tracheostomy tube in place. Other complications that can affect functional voice production, such as laryngeal stenosis or granulomas, may also result from tracheostomy tube placement. Length, as well as diameter, is also important in tube selection.

In addition to the size of the tracheostomy tube, the presence of a cuff significantly affects airflow in the upper airway. For ventilator-dependent patients in particular, an inflated cuff is typically used to maintain adequate ventilation, creating a closed system between the patient and the ventilator. The inflated cuff is also commonly used as a mechanical barrier for aspirated food or saliva, although it is well documented that cuffs do not prevent aspiration and may instead actually create physiologic and mechanical impediments to swallowing.[5-8] Tippett[9] described the drawbacks of cuff inflation as not only the loss of oral communication but also the creation of an imperfect seal against aspiration, tethering of the rise of the larynx during the swallow, and potential risk of decreased laryngeal sensitivity. Regardless of the reason the cuff is inflated, the upper airway is completely bypassed, typically creating aphonia.

Loss of airflow in the upper airway also disrupts the normal senses of olfaction and taste. These senses are dependent on the stimulation of chemoreceptor cells in the nasal mucosa, largely via airflow. With the loss of airflow into the nasal cavity, olfaction is lost. Without airflow, taste buds on the tongue also receive less stimulation. Reduction of appetite may occur with the loss of smell and taste.[10]

Loss of Subglottic Air Pressure

An unoccluded tracheostomy tube interferes with the subglottic air pressure needed for normal phonation and non-speech tasks such as effective swallowing, coughing, and defecation. Eibling and Diez-Gross[11] demonstrated that only a minimal rise in subglottic air pressure occurred in patients with open tracheostomy tubes. Individuals with open tracheostomy tubes will be unable to produce a Valsalva maneuver—the production of high intrathoracic pressure. Diez-Gross et al[12] also demonstrated potential effects of decreased subglottic air pressure in patients with unoccluded tracheostomy tubes.

Loss of the Glottic Closure Reflex

The loss of the glottic closure response and a decrease in vocal-fold mobility after tracheostomy has been reported by

several authors. Ikari and Sasaki[13] related the loss of "phasic glottic function" in the patient with a tracheostomy to changes in subglottic pressure, which consequently affects cricothyroid muscle activity, adductor function of the larynx, and glottic closure. A rise in subglottic pressure appears to be needed for a true glottic closure response to occur. Buckwalter and Sasaki[14] also noted that adductor dysfunction may contribute to failure of glottic closure, resulting in diminished cough. They stated that "adduction of the vocal cords [is] a reflex process that is most complex and therefore most vulnerable to airway alterations accompanying tracheotomy."

Blunting of the Reflexive Cough

Along with the loss of the glottic closure response, the loss of airflow through the upper airway removes the driving force of the cough, an integral mechanism for the clearing and expectoration of airway secretions. Siebens et al[8] reported that, during a cough, peak airflow velocity is increased, providing a powerful expiratory clearing force. This clearing mechanism is unavailable to individuals with an open tracheostomy tube.

Loss of Vocal-Fold Mobility

Buckwalter and Sasaki[14] reported that abductor movement of the cords is also affected in tracheostomy patients. They stated that "when spontaneous breathing is shunted through a tracheostomy, abductor activity not only gradually diminishes but disappears." The decrease in posterior cricothyroid muscle activity and abductor movement is related to the loss of intratracheal pressure.

MECHANICAL IMPACT OF TRACHEOSTOMY

Postintubation Changes

Colice[15] reported that, among a group of 54 patients who experienced prolonged translaryngeal intubation, 78% experienced laryngeal injury and hoarseness, which resolved over a period of 8 weeks. The author concluded that direct laryngoscopy should be recommended for patients whose hoarseness did not resolve within approximately 4 weeks, the median time to laryngeal re-epithelialization and healing. When healing occurs by secondary mechanisms, laryngeal granulomas may form. Persistent hoarseness indicates these more significant laryngeal injuries such as granuloma, scarring, or the formation of a posterior commissure web. These injuries can affect voice by decreasing vocal fold mobility, and may result in a reduced laryngeal airway, which also impacts normal vocal fold function. Decreased vocal fold function and reduced airway protection after prolonged orotracheal intubation is also possible.[16]

Restriction of Laryngeal Elevation

The presence of a tracheostomy is commonly felt to restrict the ability of the larynx to elevate during speech and non-speech movements. Although most reports are anecdotal, a surgical tracheotomy may restrict laryngeal elevation when the tracheostomy tube is sutured in place. Limiting the excursion of the laryngeal elevators can restrict movement of the larynx superiorly and affect lengthening of the vocal folds, one mechanism for changes in pitch. The other primary mechanism for varying pitch is the action of the cricothyroid muscle, which is known to be affected by reduced subglottic airflow and pressure.

Tracheostomy Tube Cuffs

In addition to creating aphonia, long-term tracheostomy and cuff inflation is associated with numerous potential complications. Interference with the mucosal blood supply may create eventual necrosis of tracheal cartilages, leading to possible tracheal stenosis, trachealmalacia, and, more rarely, tracheoarterial or tracheoesophageal fistula.[17,18] These complications can persist after decannulation and typically require surgical correction. Significant laryngeal injury may therefore impact both airway patency and phonation.

MECHANICAL VENTILATION: IMPACT ON COMMUNICATION

Cuff Inflation

Patients who are mechanically ventilated are commonly maintained with an inflated cuff, especially in intensive or acute care settings. Patients who are ventilator-dependent with full cuff inflation will experience aphonia and be at risk for the numerous potential complications associated with tracheostomy tube cuffs. Although alternatives to full cuff inflation for long-term ventilator-dependent patients exist, there are also many factors that impact the patient's ability to tolerate cuff deflation

Timing Issues: Coordination of Ventilation and Phonation

When a cuff is partly or fully deflated and the appropriate ventilator modifications are made, a patient may be able to produce *leak speech* around the sides of the tracheostomy tube and deflated cuff. The patient uses airflow supplied by the ventilator during the inspiratory push. Voice quality is often reduced in volume and, of necessity, syllable length.[19] It is difficult to coordinate phonation with the brief air supply given by the ventilator, and patients often find this effort tiring. Use of a one-way ventilator speaking valve, such as a Passy-Muir™, can improve the ease and quality of voice production for ventilator-dependent patients.

Mechanical Restraints of the Tube

The equipment required by ventilator-dependent patients, including tubing and humidification systems, creates additional mechanical weight on the tracheostomy tube and on the patient's larynx. In the presence of inflated cuffs ventilator-dependent patients may find it difficult to effectively elevate the larynx. If the tracheostomy tube hub is pulled downward, the end of the tube can hit the tracheal wall, causing discomfort and possibly occluding the patient's airflow. This can be influenced by both the patient's positioning and the type of tracheostomy tube used.

ORAL COMMUNICATION OPTIONS: INDICATIONS

Mouthing

Mouthing is an obvious and sometimes overlooked communication strategy. The effectiveness of mouthing is highly dependent on both the skill of the speaker and the communication partner. Only a small percentage of speech sounds are obvious on the lips, and articulatory precision and speaking rate will significantly affect intelligibility. Individuals who are aphonic can be taught to enhance their intelligibility via overarticulation and phrasing. These techniques will be most effective when mouthing is paired with another oral communication option, such as an electrolarynx.

Electrolarynges

Electrolarynges are excellent short-term communication options that can quickly facilitate communication with an aphonic patient in the intensive or acute care settings. They are easily portable, fairly simple to use, and provide an immediate source of voice. The standard, hand-held electrolarynx must be in firm contact with the patient's neck. The patient articulates while the electrolarynx provides a sound source. The artificial voice provided by the electrolarynx is then modulated into sound by the patient. The alternate sound source temporarily eliminates the need for upper-airway airflow or vocal fold vibration.

Ideal candidates for this device include aphonic patients who are attempting to mouth words, and who have fair to good articulatory control. Placement of the vibratory source varies. The standard, hand-held electrolarynx may be difficult for a tracheostomized patient who is also ventilator-dependent to use due to positioning, tubing, and the presence of the tracheostomy ties. An intraoral adapter may be used in these cases. A thin plastic tube, connected to the electrolarynx, is placed in the mouth. Tones are generated and articulated into speech. Some instruction in the coordination of articulation with an electrolarynx is usually required. Therefore, an extremely anxious individual or one with severe cognitive-linguistic deficits may not effectively use the device.

All electrolarynges require activation of on/off and volume switches. Individuals who have poor fine-motor control, quadriplegia, or are restrained will require assistance in activating the device. Switches can be adapted to facilitate independent control.

Manipulation of the Tracheostomy Tube

The SLP will gauge the ability of the patient with a tracheostomy to produce voice during an initial assessment. Ideally, the SLP will have access to the results of a laryngeal evaluation detailing the status of the patient's airway and vocal folds. This information will help in selecting the best communication option for the patient. The SLP can gain a general understanding of the patient's voice-production abilities by briefly occluding the tracheostomy tube after cuff deflation. Most patients with a tracheostomy can tolerate cuff deflation, at least for the period of the voice evaluation. The first step in the cuff-deflation process is to obtain an order from the physician. The SLP should explain the need to reestablish airflow through the upper airway for assessment of voicing ability. It is important to suction the patient properly before and during the cuff-deflation process. Typically, if the patient has had the cuff inflated for an extended period of time, secretions will be pooled on the top of the cuff. Abrupt cuff deflation "dumps" these pooled secretions into the trachea. Abrupt deflation may also

cause a patient discomfort due to coughing, a reaction to the amount of air now flowing through the glottis. The preferred protocol is to suction with the cuff inflated, reinsert the suction catheter into the tracheostomy tube, and then slowly deflate the cuff while applying suction. The patient can be given rest periods as air is slowly drawn from the cuff. Once the cuff is fully deflated, the patient may require oral suctioning to remove secretions expectorated from the pharynx.

After suctioning, some practitioners attach a manual resuscitation bag to the patient's tracheostomy tube and provide an inspiratory "push" while encouraging the patient to cough. This will help to clear pooled secretions and any aspirated material from the pharynx and larynx.

Cuff deflation may be either partial or full. When the cuff is partially deflated, the patient achieves some control over the upper airway, as evident by the initiation of voicing, coughing, or throat clearing. However, the patient will receive the most benefit, and tolerate occlusion of the tracheostomy tube optimally after full cuff deflation, so this should be a goal for the initial communication evaluation. After proper suctioning and cuff deflation, the speech-language pathologist then occludes the tracheostomy tube and assesses the patient's ability to vocalize.

Size

If the patient appears to be making an effort to phonate and no voice is heard, the size of the tracheostomy tube should be considered. A tracheostomy tube that fills more than two-thirds to three-quarters of the tracheal lumen severely restricts airflow. If possible, the patient's head can be repositioned to ensure that the tracheostomy tube is properly aligned in the trachea. If the patient remains aphonic, it will be unclear whether the cause is the size of the tracheostomy tube or actual vocal fold dysfunction. Generally, when a patient is unable to achieve any voice despite obvious efforts, the tracheostomy tube is preventing airflow from reaching the cords. A downsize of the tube can be requested from the physician, especially if the tracheostomy tube appears large relative to the size of the patient.

Type

The type of tracheostomy tube can be modified to assist the voice assessment. A fenestrated tracheostomy tube may allow voicing even in the presence of a large tube or an inflated cuff. Fenestrations may be either single or multiple. The presence of the fenestration will allow some air to reach the vocal folds (Fig 11–1). At times, the actual fenestration is situated so that it contacts the posterior tracheal wall. This is not uncommon and is, unfortunately, one cause of the granuloma formation associated with fenestrated tracheostomy tubes.[20] Many practitioners do not use fenestrated tracheostomy tubes because of the incidence of granulomas, which might eventually lead to tracheal obstruction, and tracheal bleeding upon removal of the fenestrated cannula. Multiple smaller fenestrations are designed to decrease the risk of tracheal wall irritation and granuloma formation.

The speech-language pathologist must determine if both the inner and outer cannulas of the tracheostomy tube are fenestrated. If the inner cannula is non-fenestrated, removal will reveal the fenestration or opening on the outer cannula and should allow airflow. The patient can be asked to phonate at this time. If there is a fenestrated inner cannula, it can be left in place and occluded while the patient attempts to produce voice.

A fenestrated inner cannula is available with Mallinkrodt Medical's (Tyco Healthcare) tracheostomy tubes and is identified by a green tip. It is interchangeable with the nonfenestrated cannula, which can be used if a patient is ventilator-dependent part of the day.

If the patient is still unable to achieve voice after cuff deflation, positioning changes, and tracheostomy tube modifications, vocal fold dysfunction should be suspected and a direct laryngeal examination by an otolaryngologist would be recommended.

Specialty Tracheostomy Tubes

Some patients with special airway needs require tracheostomy tubes with specific features such as additional length. Specialty tracheostomy tubes compensate for

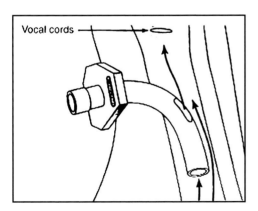

Fig 11–1. Airflow moving through a fenestration (cuffless, fenestrated tracheostomy tube). From Dikeman and Kazandjian.[19] Reproduced with permission.

anatomic abnormalities which can not be addressed with the length, material, or design of a standard tube. Figure 11-2 depicts an extra-long specialty tracheostomy tube.

Cuff Deflation

Cuff deflation offers numerous advantages to the patient with a tracheostomy, one of which may be the ability to achieve phonation. As noted, most patients with a tracheostomy can tolerate cuff deflation for at least the duration of the voice evaluation. Some patients in the process of being weaned from the ventilator and receiving high levels of oxygen may need the inflated cuff to maintain oxygenation. Cuffs can also assist in reducing (although not preventing) aspiration of secretions. Individuals with copious secretions may require the mechanical barrier of the inflated cuff to assist in airway protection. Therefore, medical clearance and individual patient assessment—usually by the physician, nurse, respiratory care practitioner, and speech pathologist is recommended prior to cuff deflation.

Full or at least partial deflation is recommended to normalize airflow in the upper airway and restore phonation and airway protection abilities. When the tracheostomy tube is properly sized and the cuff is deflated, a patient with adequate vocal fold function should produce voice

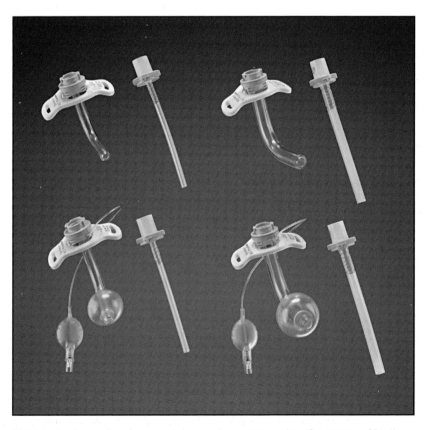

Fig 11–2. Example of a specialty tracheostomy tube. Courtesy of Nellcor.

upon tracheal occlusion. Although finger occlusion is helpful during the initial assessment and is useful for medical staff to obtain quick responses from the patient, its ongoing use for communication purposes is not recommended. Finger occlusion is often difficult for patients to coordinate, is a potential source of infection, and does not provide the consistent closed system that promotes restoration of normal airway responses. Any patient with an unoccluded tracheostomy tube in place for more than a few days, and who meets specific criteria, should be assessed for use of a one-way speaking valve.

One-Way Speaking Valves

One-way tracheostomy speaking valves are removable devices that are placed on the 15-mm hub of the tracheostomy tube, either the inner or outer cannula, eliminating the need for finger occlusion to achieve voice. One-way valves serve to redirect airflow through the tracheostomy tube to the vocal folds by allowing air to enter the tracheostomy tube upon inspiration. Upon expiration, the valve is closed, and air is redirected through the upper airway instead of back through the tracheostomy tube. Closure mechanisms differ dependent on the type of valve being used. Voice is produced on expiration as air vibrates the vocal folds and flows through the oral and nasal cavities, creating a normalized pattern for the patient. The patient is able to inspire through the tracheostomy tube, bypassing the resistance of the upper airway, but regains the benefit of voicing upon expiration and using the upper airway.

One-way tracheostomy speaking valves provide varying degrees of airway resist-

ance. Careful patient assessment is necessary prior to use. This assessment must include both the patient's pulmonary and airway status. The patient must be able to exhale sufficient amounts of air, optimally the same amount inhaled, around the sides of the tracheostomy tube and deflated cuff. Failure to ensure adequate airflow out through the upper airway can lead to eventual barotrauma of the lungs and serious pulmonary consequences. General candidacy for use of a speaking valve includes the factors outlined below.

Ability to Tolerate Cuff Deflation

Adequate exhalation through the upper airway is essential for the use of a speaking valve. The patient can no longer exhale out through the tracheostomy tube with the one-way valve in place. Pressure in the airway and lungs will increase quickly, and the patient will not be able to inspire. Insufficient air exchange and eventually barotrauma can result. Cuff deflation is mandatory for the successful use of a speaking valve. For this reason, tracheostomy tubes with foam cuffs are contraindicated with one-way speaking valves, as they may reinflate in the trachea.

Ability to Produce Voice upon Tracheal (Finger) Occlusion

The ability to phonate with tracheal occlusion is an initial indication of adequate vocal fold function and the ability to move air around the sides of the tracheostomy tube. Because of the additional resistance of inspired air created by the speaking valve, and the need to exhale around the tube out through the upper airway, the tracheostomy tube may be downsized to allow extended speaking valve use.

Maintenance of Acceptable Baseline Respiratory Status on Valve Placement

All one-way valves create various degrees of additional resistance to inspired air and may increase the patient's work of breathing, or effort required to maintain respiration. The patient must present with a stable respiratory status prior to intervention. Monitoring with noninvasive techniques such as pulse oximetry and capnography is useful to assess trends in oxygen saturation and carbon dioxide levels. Objective monitoring tools are paired with clinical assessment of the patient's phonation, respiratory rate, general condition, and comfort. In the absence of noninvasive monitoring tools, clinical assessment can be paired with blood gases, which should be taken after an initial trial wear period. Speaking valve wear time can be increased as tolerated. A sample protocol for placement of a one-way speaking valve is provided in Table 11–1.

Table 11–1. Sample Interdisciplinary Speaking Valve Placement Protocol for Patients with a Tracheostomy

1. Follow cuff deflation protocol, ensuring that cuff is completely deflated.
2. Place the speaking valve on the 15-mm hub of the tracheostomy tube (RT/RN/SLP).
3. If applicable, reconnect T-piece or tracheostomy collar (RT/RN/SLP).
4. Instruct patient to breathe through the upper airway by blowing out of the mouth and nose.
5. Begin trial attempts at phonation. SLP encourages patient to vocalize /ah/, count to 5, or sing a song (automatic speech tasks are especially helpful for cognitively impaired patients).
6. Simultaneously monitor O_2 saturation and CO_2 levels via oximetry and capnography (RT/RN).
7. Look for symptoms of increased work of breathing or clinical symptoms/complaints of discomfort.
8. If voice is minimal or strained, reassess breathing pattern and provide instruction in coordination of phonation with expiratory phase of respiration (eg, additional phonatory tasks such as counting and extended vowel productions coupled with assistance in diaphragmatic support) (SLP). Remember that patients may have difficulty adjusting to more normalized airflow.
9. Team will determine extent of wearing time based on results of noninvasive and invasive (ie, blood gases) monitoring and patient's clinical response to the speaking valve (MD/RN/RT/SLP).
10. Orders for speaking valve use added to patient's treatment sheet (MD).

RT, respiratory therapist; RN, registered nurse; SLP, speech-language pathologist.
Source: From Dikeman and Kazandjian.[19] Reprinted with permission from Delmar-Thomson Learning.

Speaking valves can be used for patients who receive humidification or oxygen, whether by tracheostomy collar or T-piece. Patients who receive oxygen or humidity should continue to do so while wearing a speaking valve. In fact, increased levels of O_2 or humidity may be indicated. Oxygen adapters are available with the Passy-Muir 2000 and 2001 speaking valves, with the Nellcor Phonate one-way speaking valve, and with the Boston Medical Tracoe Phon Assist I speech valve. Examples are pictured in Figures 11–3A and 11–3B. Table 11–2 summarizes commonly used speaking valves and their characteristics.

Contraindications

General contraindications for the use of a one-way speaking valve include (1) inability to tolerate cuff deflation, (2) significant airway obstruction, (3) end-stage pulmonary disease, (4) hemodynamic instability, (5) total laryngectomy, and (6) anarthria (severe motor-speech impairment). Patients with poor pulmonary function often exhibit carbon dioxide retention and may also have difficulty tolerating a one-way speaking valve. Some degree of air trapping does occur with valve placement, and individuals with overly compliant lungs may not fully exhale. Elevated CO_2 levels can result, and should be carefully monitored. As noted, capnography is an effective tool to detect rising CO_2 levels. Patients who are hemodynamically unstable are less likely to tolerate the potential increase in work of breathing created by the speaking valve.

Although one-way speaking valves will not restore oral communication abilities to individuals with anarthria or severe dysarthria, studies have addressed other benefits of one-way valves. For example, the literature describes the specific use of the Passy-Muir™ valve for improved swallowing and reduction of aspiration[21-23] to facilitate decannulation[24,25] and for improved olfaction and secretion management.[26]

Types of Speaking Valves

Tracheostomy speaking valves can be classified into two types, open- and closed-position. These terms refer to the

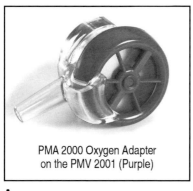

PMA 2000 Oxygen Adapter
on the PMV 2001 (Purple)

A.

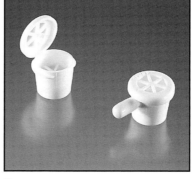

B.

Fig 11–3. A. The Passy-Muir 2001 tracheostomy and ventilator one-way speaking valve with oxygen adapter; Courtesy of Passy-Muir, Inc. **B.** The Shiley/Mallinkrodt Phonate tracheostomy speaking valve; Photo courtesy of Nellcor.

Table 11–2. Selected Speaking Valves and Their Characteristics

Valve	Type	Attachment to Trachs	Valve Characteristics
Passy-Muir speaking valve, Passy-Muir, Inc.	One-way valve (closed position); different valves available for tracheostomized and/or ventilator-dependent individuals	Fits on 15-mm hub of tracheostomy tube or can be placed in line with ventilator tubing	One-way Silastic membrane with bias closed position, opens upon inspiration, creating a "positive closure" feature. Low profile design/color and oxygen port and adapter available
Montgomery tracheostomy speaking valve, Boston Medical Products	One-way valve	Fits 15-mm hub of tracheostomy tube	Silicone membrane is hinged; maintains open position but opens more fully upon inspiration. Cough release feature
VentTrach speaking valve, Boston Medical Products	One-way valve	Fits 15-mm hub of tracheostomy tube	Approved for use with ventilator-dependent as well as tracheostomized patients, valve closes to decrease backflow from expired air
Tracheo® Phon Assist 1 Speech Valve, Boston Medical Products	One-way valve	Fits 15-mm hub of tracheostomy tube	Adjustable airflow feature sets resistance to expired air; oxygen port available
Phonate Speaking Valve, Nellcor	One-way valve	Fits 15-mm hub of tracheostomy tube	Hinged cap for cleaning valve membrane, oxygen supplement port and cap available
Hood Speaking Valve, Hood Laboratories	One-way valve	Fits 15-mm hub of tracheostomy tube	Available for tracheostomy tubes and other anesthesia devices; specify type wanted when ordering
Medin Low Resistance Speaking Valve, Hood Laboratories	One-way valve	Fits 15-mm hub of tracheostomy tube	Available for tracheostomy tubes and other anesthesia devices; specify type wanted when ordering
Eliachaer Speaking Valve, Hood Laboratories	One-way valve	For use with Hood stoma stents	Flap design, low resistance, low profile speaking valve for use with Hood stoma stents.

resting position of the one-way membrane that allows passage of air into the tracheostomy tube during inspiration. Open-position valves, as the name implies, maintain an open "set," opening further on the push of inspired air. The valve mechanism is pushed closed during expiration. A small amount of air leakage does occur back out of the tracheotomy tube at this time. Most one-way tracheostomy valves fall into this general category. The only closed-position valve currently on the market is the Passy-Muir™. This valve contains a Silastic membrane that retains its closed position against the front of the valve until inspiration. On inspiration, the valve opens; then it closes automatically at the end of expiration. The company describes this feature, which prevents air leakage out the valve, as "positive closure." The positive closure feature appears to facilitate other benefits described in the literature with regard to use of the Passy-Muir speaking valve, especially in terms of increased subglottic air pressures and in some instances, improved swallowing.[12]

One-way speaking valves should be considered for most tracheostomized patients. Benefits include elimination of finger occlusion, facilitation of voicing, normalization of airflow, and assistance with weaning and decannulation. One-way valves are an effective interim step in the tracheostomy weaning process.

Cannula Systems

Specially designed cannula systems, which may take the place of a tracheostomy tube and serve to maintain an open stoma, can facilitate oral communication when paired with plugs or speaking valves. One example is the Boston Medical Products Traceo® long-term cannula system. When using a plug or button, a patient must rely completely on the upper airway for respiration. A one-way valve allows use of the cannula for breathing. Cannula systems are useful in weaning the patient from a tracheostomy tube.

Alternatively, Eliachar[27] used a surgical option to construct a tube-free stoma which permitted unaided speech production and an effective cough. The long-term flap procedure was successful for a number of long-term tracheostomy patients who met specific selection criteria. These included alert, motivated individuals without neuromuscular or head and neck conditions and diseases.

Special Considerations: Ventilator-Dependent Patients

The restoration of oral communication to the ventilator-dependent patient may involve manipulation of both the tracheostomy tube and the settings of the ventilator. These ventilator modifications always involve the respiratory therapist and, in some settings, the nurse. For the speech-language pathologist, the same initial assessment of articulatory and phonatory abilities used with the tracheostomized individual is necessary. However, the initial step in the evaluation process must be deflation of the tracheostomy tube cuff. Most ventilator-dependent patients are maintained with the cuff inflated to insure that they receive the tidal volume being delivered from the ventilator. The cuff compensates for the area in the tracheal lumen that is not filled by the tracheostomy tube itself. When the cuff is deflated, air can escape around the sides of the tracheostomy tube and out the upper airway. Although this escape of air out of the upper airway has positive implications for speech (and potentially swallowing), it does affect delivered tidal volume. Ventilator modifications are usually necessary to compensate for the volume leak created by deflating the cuff. The use of cuff deflation with ventilator-dependent patients has been reported by a number of practitioners, including Dikeman and Kazandjian,[19] Bach and Alba,[28] Tippett and Siebens,[29] Manzano et al,[30] Kazandjian et al,[31] and Conway and Mackie.[32]

Tippett[9] maintained ventilator settings during cuff deflation by modifying the positioning of the patient and allowing the velum and tongue to approximate the posterior pharyngeal wall, modulating airway resistance. Tippett and Siebens[29] described the use of glottic control, or volitional use of the vocal folds to regulate airflow through the upper airway— as a technique to allow cuff deflation. Ventilation with cuff deflation is possible, even at night, with these techniques. More commonly, adjustments of the ventilator can be made on an individual basis to compensate for the loss of air created by cuff deflation. These adjustments usually involve a change, usually an increase, in the tidal volume set on the ventilator. For example, if the patient should receive a tidal volume of 800 mL and the tracheostomy tube cuff is deflated, the volume that the patient receives, and is registered by the exhaled tidal volume alarm, will decrease. This decrease may be 200 mL or more and can be measured at the mouth by a spirometer with an oral adapter. The respiratory therapist can compensate for the leak by gradually increasing the tidal volume set on the ventilator to 200 mL above the original

setting used with the inflated cuff. The goal is adequate ventilation with the preservation of phonation. Care must be taken to make sure that excessive tidal volumes are not used. This is accomplished by a slow increase in tidal volume, careful assessment of the high-pressure alarms on the ventilator, and ongoing noninvasive and clinical monitoring.

Respiratory rate and the inspiratory/ expiratory ratio are two additional settings that are commonly adjusted by the respiratory therapist to help the patient tolerate cuff deflation. When a patient is using "*leak speech*," (the term used to describe phonation with cuff deflation) speech takes place on the inspiratory cycle of the ventilator. It is at this point in the ventilatory cycle that air is available for phonation. Adjusting (often decreasing) the ventilatory rate, and/or lengthening the inspiratory phase of the inspiratory:expiratory ratio may give the patient more time to phonate. It is the primary role of the respiratory therapist to assess a patient's ability to tolerate these ventilator modifications and remain adequately ventilated, although the entire team will be involved in ongoing, daily clinical assessment. Again, noninvasive monitoring tools such as pulse oximetry and capnography are extremely valuable in ongoing patient monitoring.

One-Way Valves

The use of a one-way tracheostomy speaking valve in line with ventilator tubing can enhance oral communication significantly. The Passy-Muir™ and the Ventrach™ (Boston Medical Products) are the only one-way speaking valves with FDA approval for in-line ventilator use. At this time, the Passy-Muir™ closed-position speaking valve has been used most extensively with ventilator-dependent patients, with applications for communication, weaning, and swallowing reported throughout the literature.[30,33-35] Because of the positive closure feature of the Passy-Muir valve, there is no air leakage back into the tracheostomy tube and ventilatory circuitry. This ensures that, when ventilator modifications are made, all of the ventilator volume will be delivered to the patient. Additionally, air that accumulates in the tracheostomy tube and in the airway is available for phonation regardless of the cycle of the ventilator. To avoid excessive air trapping, especially with patients with diseased lungs, tidal volume and high-pressure alarms must be carefully monitored. The upper airway must be free of any obstruction; complete cuff deflation and optimal tracheotomy tube size relative to the patient's tracheal lumen are critical. The Passy-Muir 007 ventilator valve is pictured in Figure 11-4.

Ventilator alarms are a consideration. With a valve in place, air will not return to the ventilator, and the exhaled tidal volume alarm will consequently sound.

This is often unsettling to patients and staff. Collaboration with the respiratory therapist is essential to complete ventilator modifications that allow in-line speaking valve use.

The transdisciplinary team concept is essential for a successful in-line ventilator speaking valve placement. The initial use of the valve is assessed by speech pathology, respiratory care, and nursing. A baseline respiratory status should be obtained, and the patient must be monitored throughout the initial wear period. A sample protocol for a transdisciplinary speaking valve placement (Passy-Muir) with a ventilator-dependent patient is provided in Table 11-3. Further protocols for speaking valve placement are available in the literature,[19] and through Passy-Muir, Inc.

Talking Tracheostomy Tubes

Talking or "speaking" tracheostomy tubes are indicated primarily for patients who are candidates for oral communication but cannot tolerate cuff deflation. This specialized tracheostomy tube is constructed with an external line for connection to a separate air source, such as humidified air. Inside the tracheostomy tube, there is an outlet for the air in the trachea, above the level of the cuff. The airflow from the separate air source is regulated by a port on the external line, as pictured in Figure 11-5. When the port is covered, air is directed into the trachea. When it is open, air escapes into the atmosphere. This avoids a constant source of airflow, which might be irritating to the laryngeal mucosa.

Talking tracheostomy tubes are available in a number of designs and materials, including single or multiple fenestrations,

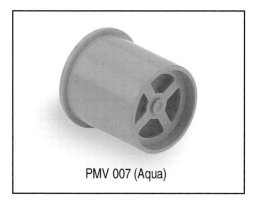

PMV 007 (Aqua)

Fig 11-4. The Passy-Muir 007 one-way ventilator (and tracheostomy) speaking valve. Photo courtesy of Passy-Muir, Inc.

Table 11–3. Sample Interdisciplinary Speaking Valve Placement Protocol for Ventilator-Dependent Patients

1. Begin with the suctioning and cuff deflation protocol (MD/RT/RN/SLP).

2. Ensure total cuff deflation with appropriate ventilator modifications (eg, increase tidal volume setting) (RT). Monitor closely while allowing for "leak speech."

3. Place the speaking valve on the hub of the patient's tracheostomy tube. The speaking valve can then be connected to a section of disposable tubing which attaches to the ventilator tubing (RT/RN/SLP). (Recall that the need for an additional section of tubing to be used as an adapter will depend on the individual setup (where the valve is being placed in the ventilator circuitry). The valve may also be placed upon the swivel adapter of the ventilator.

4. Readjust the exhaled tidal volume alarm (RT).

5. Watch the response of the ventilator and monitoring tools after introduction of the valve. Observe the peak inspiratory pressure, respiratory rate, heart rate, oxygen saturation, and carbon dioxide levels (RT/RN). Readjust the ventilator settings (eg, increase or decrease tidal volume) as needed (RT).

6. SLP instructs patient in usage of the upper airway via "blowing out" air through vocalization, singing, counting, or conversation. Use of bedside spirometry may also facilitate relearning upper airway usage. Remind the patient that talking is possible throughout the ventilator cycle.

7. Utilize additional ventilator modifications as needed: pressure support, increased FiO_2, respiratory rate, sensitivity setting (RT). As long as the patient is not in distress, explore these changes to enhance patient's voice and comfort.

8. Determine if patient can tolerate a consistent wear schedule. Assign team members responsibilities for valve use according to facility policy and procedure.

9. Following valve use, detach the valve from tracheostomy tube hub and reconnect swivel adapter in-line. Readjust ventilator settings and alarms to previous levels (RT). Reinflate cuff if patient has not been tolerating long-term cuff deflation.

10. Team assesses patient's ability to tolerate cuff deflation and Passy-Muir speaking valve usage (MD/RT/RN/SLP).

11. Order for speaking valve use placed on patient's treatment schedule.

RT, respiratory therapist; RN, registered nurse; SLP, speech-language pathologist.
Source: From Dikeman and Kazandjian.[19] Reproduced with permission from Delmar-Thomson Learning.

foam cuffs, and silicone tubes. Figure 11–6 illustrates Bivona Fome-Cuf™ and Aire-Cuf™ with talk attachment. Nomori[36] designed and reported the use of a "voice tracheostomy tube" which enabled cuff inflation upon inspired positive pressure

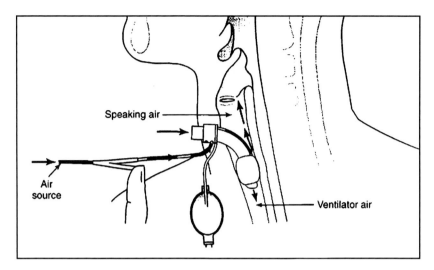

Fig 11–5. A "talking" tracheostomy tube, with the external port occluded to allow phonation. From Dikeman and Kazandjian.[19] Reproduced with permission.

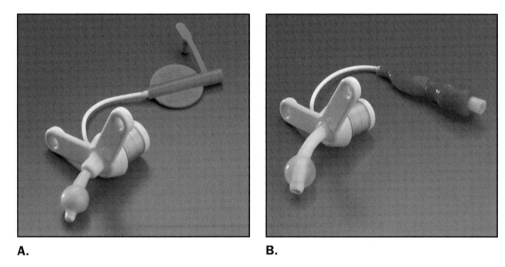

A.   **B.**

Fig 11–6. The Bivona Fome-Cuf (**A**) and Aire-Cuf (**B**) speaking tracheostomy tubes. Photo courtesy of Bivona Medical Technologies.

from a ventilator, and cuff deflation upon expiration. This allowed inspired air from the ventilator to pass around the deflated cuff and permit vocalization.

As noted, a talking tracheostomy tube is an oral communication option for a patient who cannot tolerate cuff deflation. Candidates must have adequate articulation, as the talking tracheostomy tube provides only air for phonation. Typical users of talking tracheostomy tubes include medically fragile patients or those with advanced pulmonary disease.

Issues for functional use of a talking tracheostomy tube usually include speech intelligibility. The airflow must typically be adjusted before the patient achieves a functional voice, usually beginning with a flow of at least 6 L/min and progressing to 12 L/min to 15 L/min. Humidification of the air source is important to avoid drying of laryngeal tissues.

Leder[37] discussed prognostic variables for successful use of a talking tracheostomy tube. These included stable medical status, daily practice and intervention with the device, proper airflow adjustment, adequate oromotor skills, and user motivation. Careful patient selection will increase the chance of success with a talking tracheostomy tube.[19]

The use of a talking tracheostomy tube also dictates a careful, transdiscipli-nary protocol. A sample is provided in Table 11–4. Talking tracheostomy tubes should be considered for any patient with the potential for restoration of vocal communication.

NONORAL COMMUNICATION OPTIONS: INDICATIONS

Restoring vocal or oral communication is an important goal following tracheostomy. However, for some patients, voice or speech production is not possible either for temporary or extended time periods. During this "nonoral" period,

Table 11–4. Sample Interdisciplinary "Talking" Tracheostomy Tube Placement Protocol

1. Placement of the talking tracheostomy tube is accomplished with the members of the interdisciplinary team during a routine tracheostomy tube change (MD/RT/RN). It is optional to wait 24 hours to allow any edema to subside before attempting voice production.

2. Suction the patient following the established suctioning procedure to lessen the chance of pooled secretions blocking the airflow outlets (RT/RN/SLP).

3. Determine the source of external air. Attach the external airflow line to the air source. Connect a source of humidification (RT) to the tracheostomy.

4. Regulate airflow as the patient is encouraged to vocalize. Begin with approximately 6 L/min and adjust airflow as needed in 1-L increments. (Airflow should not exceed 15 L.) Clinical judgment and patient comfort will guide this setting.

5. Continue trial attempts at phonation. Provide patient with directions to maximize speech intelligibility, such as decreasing speech rate and using overarticulation (SLP).

6. In-service patient, staff, and family in use and maintenance of the device.

7. Incorporate problem-solving methods if voice is not achieved.

8. Set a schedule for daily usage as per patient need and tolerance.

9. Request order for use of a talking tracheostomy tube from MD; place on patient's treatment sheet.

RT, respiratory therapist; RN, registered nurse; SLP speech-language pathologist.
Source: From Dikeman and Kazandjian.[19] Reproduced with permission from Delmar-Thomson Learning.

communication must continue. The term nonoral refers to a patient's inability to communicate through speech and/or voice. When oral communication is not feasible, the speech-language pathologist provides alternate options to meet daily communicative needs. Nonoral communication methods may also supplement or "augment" attempts at oral communication. Mouthing is one example. A patient can use an alphabet board to simultaneously point to the letters on the board while mouthing letters and words, clarifying attempts at oral communication. When oral attempts are unsuccessful, alternative communication options are then explored. The appropriateness of one option over another for an individual is a function of his or her current physical-motor and cognitive status, as well as the anticipated length of time for use of the nonoral communication method.

Physical Motor Status

Physical motor ability can change as the patient with a tracheostomy moves from an acute to a more stable medical status. When physical motor status is compromised, the medical team must consider alternative methods of accessing the augmentative or alternative communication system. For example, the medical team may be forced to restrain the patient with a fresh tracheostomy who has good upper extremity function but unknowingly pulls out his or her tracheostomy tube. In other situations, the tracheostomy patient may present with a medical condition that impairs motor function and consequently limits consistent, reliable movements of the upper extremity. Pointing, the obvious method of accessing a communication system, may not be possible in these cases. The key to suc-

cessful message transfer is identifying an easy-to-use, reliable, and consistent motor movement. Once residual movement is identified and selected, methods of alternative access can be explored.

The term *access* refers to the method by which the tracheostomy patient will operate the communication system. If direct selection (ie, pointing) of an item or letter is not possible, a less complex or strenuous motor movement may be available. Scanning is an example of an access method that requires less motor movement. It involves presenting items or letters until the patient uses a predetermined signal, such as looking upward, to indicate that the target has been reached. Figure 11–7 illustrates the use of row-column scanning. The patient uses established *yes* and *no* signals to indicate when the communication partner has pointed to the desired letter. The communication partner begins by pointing to the first row of letters and proceeds downward until the row containing the patient's target letter is reached. The patient signals a *yes* response. Now knowing the row, the communication partner then points to each letter along the column until the target letter is identified. If an accurate *yes/no* signal cannot be obtained by a body movement, such as a head shake or nod, a switch can be provided for clarification. Switches range in size, shape, texture, sensitivity, and complexity. The patient's residual motor movement and medical condition will determine what switch is most appropriate. Switches can be accessed by light touch or gross body movements. A speech pathologist in conjunction with an occupational therapist and rehabilitation engineer can recommend and/or fabricate a switch that can be consistently accessed by the nonoral communicator with a tracheostomy.

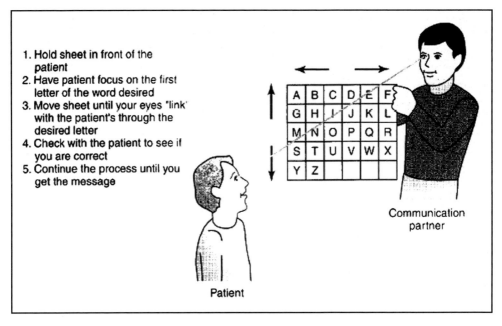

1. Hold sheet in front of the patient
2. Have patient focus on the first letter of the word desired
3. Move sheet until your eyes "link" with the patient's through the desired letter
4. Check with the patient to see if you are correct
5. Continue the process until you get the message

Communication partner

Patient

Fig 11–7. Row-column scanning. From Dikeman and Kazandjian.[19] Reproduced with permission.

Immediate Intervention

Intervention techniques for augmenting or providing alternative communication options may be immediate, short-term, or long-term.

It is not uncommon to find an alert, intubated patient with a recent tracheotomy in the medical intensive care unit without a means of expressing basic needs. In this setting, the patient's primary need is to call for assistance. As calling out for help verbally is not possible, an alternative call method must be provided. Most hospitals provide standard nursing call buzzers at the patient's bedside to alert the staff in an emergency or when attention is needed. This standard device, pictured in Figure 11–8, is usually sufficient when physical motor function is not impaired. However, patients who are temporarily restrained or exhibit upper extremity weakness often cannot access the standard call buzzer and are left with no means of immediate communication. The medical team must assess the patient's physical motor function for a consistent and reliable motor movement. For a patient with quadriplegia, this may be merely a twitch of the cheek or a slight movement of the head. Once the residual motor movement is identified, the medical team can use an alternative device for alerting or calling. Alternatives to standard nursing call buzzers include adaptive switches that are plugged directly into the bedside call system, or switches that connect to independent buzzer boxes. These buzzers activate when the switch is engaged, and can be amplified to insure that the staff easily hear the signals.

Once the aphonic patient with a tracheostomy has alerted or gained the attention of a conversational partner, clarification of the message becomes necessary. A consistent, reliable *yes/no*

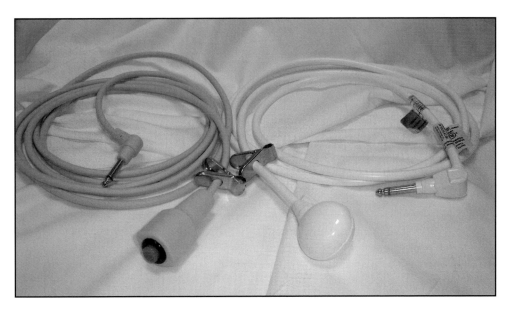

Fig 11–8. Standard call buzzers, From Dikeman and Kazandjian.[19] Reproduced with permission.

system is essential in ensuring that the exchange is a success. A *yes/no* system can take many forms, depending on the current physical motor status of the patient. When head movement is possible, head nods and shakes are most easily understood by any conversational partner. However, when motor movements of the head are restricted, an alternative system can easily be provided. Mounting the words *yes* and *no* on cards and instructing the aphonic patient to look at the desired response is often successful. Whatever system has been selected for use, basic instructions for use should be placed at bedside for all visitors and staff. Sample instructions are provided in Table 11–5. Facilitation of basic message exchange allows the patient with a tracheostomy to feel less anxious and enjoy an improved quality of life while he or she is unable to communicate verbally. The medical team can now make sure that the patient is a member of the team.

Table 11–5. Communicating with Hilda

1. Hilda uses her eyes to communicate yes or no.

2. Hold the "yes" and "no" cards separately.

3. Phrase your question so Hilda can respond with yes or no.

4. Hilda will look or stare to the left for "yes" and to the right for "no."

Short-Term Intervention

Although immediate intervention techniques are necessary for all nonspeaking patients with a tracheostomy, short-term intervention allows for the expression of messages with more detail. Once the attention of a conversational partner has been gained, short-term techniques allow patient with a tracheostomy to ask questions or make detailed comments. These short-term systems include writing, communication boards, and other "low-tech" devices.

Writing is the most readily available and portable communication system. When the patient has fine motor movement available, he or she can be provided with a pen and pad of paper, a magnetic board, or a "Magic Slate." With this reusable board, messages can be easily erased by lifting the top sheet. These inexpensive items can be purchased in toy or stationery stores. When upper extremity movement is reduced, writing may still be possible with adaptive devices for positioning and better control. They can be provided by an occupational therapist.

Communication boards can take many forms depending on the patient's cognitive communication status as well as his or her physical motor ability. Alphabet boards, phrase/word boards, and picture boards are all useful in transferring pertinent messages and clarifying ideas and requests. The speech-language pathologist will assess the patient's overall language ability before determining what type of communication board is appropriate. The goal of fabricating a communication board is to provide the most time-efficient, functional system facilitating accurate message transfer. A word/phrase board can be combined with an alphabet board to allow for quick and easy message exchange as well as an opportunity for clarification and detail. For example, a communication board can be created with two sides, one with the alphabet and one with frequently used words and phrases such as "Thank you" and "Please suction me."

When physical motor function is severely limited but eye movement remains reliable, the use of an Eye-Link[38] to directly select and spell messages is very helpful. Figure 11–9 illustrates the use of an Eye-Link as the patient uses eye gaze to select the desired letters of an alphabet board through a sheet of transparent plastic. Only eye movement is required from the patient; however, movement of the extremities is necessary from the conversational partner. The patient stares directly at the target letter. The Eye-Link is moved up and down, side to side in front of the patient until the patient's eye gaze "links" with the eye gaze of the conversational partner. This indicates the selected item. The Eye-Link has been used successfully in a wide variety of settings with nonoral adults with tracheostomies, who were also ventilator-dependent.[30]

When there is a need for more sophisticated communication methods, for example, telephone exchanges or hardcopy printout messages, more "high-tech" systems may be introduced. Electronic communication devices (Fig 11–10) can provide the patient with a tracheostomy in the acute care setting with both synthesized voice output and hardcopy printout. Printed messages can be prepared by the patient prior to contact with members of the medical team. This time efficient method is often helpful in a busy acute care environment, for example, to prepare a question for a physician.

Long-Term Intervention

Short-term solutions are often sufficient for patients who may regain oral communication abilities. However, some patients with tracheostomies present with medical conditions that may deteriorate over time (ie, amyotrophic lateral sclerosis) or that leave them permanently nonspeaking

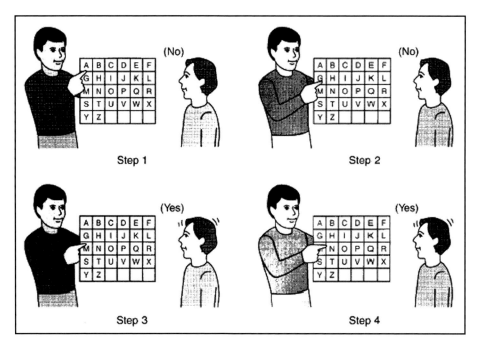

Fig 11–9. An eye-link communication system in use. From Dikeman and Kazandjian.[19] Reproduced with permission.

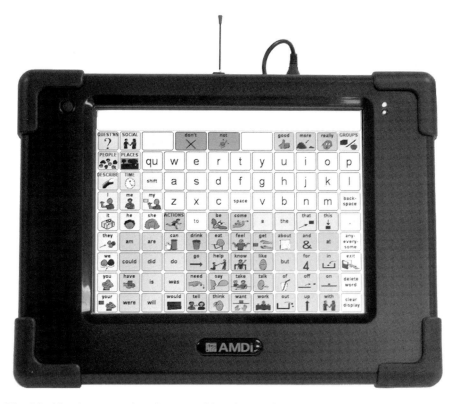

Fig 11–10. An example of a portable electronic communication device. Photo courtesy of AMDi.

(ie, brainstem cerebrovascular accident). They require long-term communication options. These long-term solutions are often referred to as "high-tech" devices. Such electronic devices—often with computer capability, hard-copy printout, speech synthesis, and modem access—allow the patient with a tracheostomy to communicate on sophisticated terms in the widest variety of settings. High-tech alternative communication systems also provide increased independence, as the patient can access preprogrammed utterances for rate-enhancement purposes during conversational exchange. For example, the phrase "suction me" can be accessed by use of two letters on a keyboard, such as "SM." With high-tech solutions, patients may communicate via a computer modem on-line, expanding the opportunity for information access through the Internet and E-mail communication. Even when physical motor movements are significantly limited, as in quadriplegic patients, switch access combined with sophisticated computer capability can allow the patient with a tracheotomy to prepare and communicate novel utterances verbally, through a speech synthesizer, and on paper with a printer.

The following case vignette follows one patient with a tracheostomy through a course of nonoral and oral communication intervention.

CASE VIGNETTE

Days 1 to 30

Joe, a 77-year-old man, was admitted to the cardiac critical care unit intubated and ventilator-dependent following cardiac bypass graft surgery. Medical diag-noses included cardiac vessel disease, previous angioplasty, congestive heart failure, and respiratory failure. Ventilator weaning attempts after surgery over the next 18 days were unsuccessful due to medical complications, including pneumonia. A tracheotomy was performed on the 18th postoperative day. A No. 8 cuffed nonfenestrated tracheostomy tube was placed. A nasogastric tube had been placed for nutrition and hydration, and was replaced by a percutaneous jejunostomy tube on day 21. Full support from the ventilator and a fully inflated tracheostomy tube cuff were required. Joe's decreased cognitive communication status and decreased level of alertness in the weeks immediately following the procedure limited his ability to communicate by either oral or nonoral methods. On day 30, he became more alert for short periods. He began to mouth rapidly, with little regard for his conversational partner's comprehension. Confusion was apparent throughout the day and night as he continually pulled the ventilator tubing off his tracheostomy tube, despite verbal reminders from medical staff and his family. Restraints became necessary to prevent disconnection from the ventilator. Joe's attempts at writing, with the restraints briefly removed, were illegible. By day 34 post surgery, the patient became more consistently alert and awake, and more purposeful attempts at communication were noted by staff. A speech-language pathology consultation was requested.

Day 34

On initial evaluation, Joe did not have an effective means of message transfer. This frustrated not only him but also his family and the medical team. Intervention was directed at providing Joe with an immediate method of message transfer. The medical staff had made sure that Joe could access the nursing call buzzer despite his physical restraints. However, once Joe had used the call buzzer and the nurse entered the room, a breakdown in communication occurred; therefore a *yes/no* communication system was devised. Directions for use were placed above Joe's bed. This ensured that all people entering the room were aware of Joe's inability to communicate verbally, and provided simple instructions for message transfer. Head movements were not completely reliable, but Joe was able to "look up for yes." The communication partner would remind him of the directions prior to asking him a question, and then observe his response. As Joe became more alert and less restless, he was able to access a letter/word/phrase board via pointing to convey simple requests to staff and family. More functional mouthing was also noted.

Day 36

By day 36, the acute pneumonia had resolved and Joe's medical status was stable. Ventilator weaning efforts were initiated by the medical team. Occasionally Joe's voice could be heard when he mouthed words. He appeared ready to use an oral communication method. The speech-language pathologist requested an order for cuff deflation for voice assessment. Once the order was obtained, the respiratory therapist and speech pathologist came to the bedside together for the assessment. The patient was receiving control mode ventilation with a rate of 10 and a tidal volume of 800 mL.

The cuff was gradually deflated to the point at which efforts at phonation were audible. As Joe became accustomed to the airflow through the upper airway, more air was gradually removed from the cuff until it was fully deflated. He exhibited some reaction to the airflow through the upper airway, as evident by coughing. He was assisted in the transition process with instructions to vocalize and exhale out the nose and mouth. Ventilator settings were modified by the respiratory therapist. Tidal volume was increased 150 mL and pressure-support ventilation was added. Joe's vocal quality was significantly dysphonic. An otolaryngology consultation was requested.

Day 37

The direct fiberoptic assessment, conducted with partial cuff deflation, revealed that both vocal folds were mobile. No granulomas or other lesions were noted. Joe was noted to aspirate his own secretions during the assessment, and demonstrated poor coughing and secretion clearance.

Days 38 to 42

On day 38 Joe was transferred to a subacute facility with a specialized tracheostomy and ventilator unit. Weaning attempts continued. He was changed to synchronized intermittent mandatory ventilation (SIMV) with a rate of 8. By day 42, he tolerated continuous positive airway pressure (CPAP) for several hours during the day and received SIMV at night. With speech pathology and respiratory therapy assistance, periods of cuff deflation for oral communication and restoration of upper airway function continued. The patient was encouraged to swallow his own saliva and use an intermittent cough/throat clear after the swallow. A Passy-Muir™ speaking valve placement was completed on day 41; the patient tolerated the in-line valve for short periods. A schedule of 30-minute wear intervals was set with respiratory therapy and nursing, and a flow chart for tracking valve use was placed at the bedside.

Day 43

In order to assess swallowing function and any potential for p.o. intake, a videofluoroscopy was performed. During the examination, the patient was ventilator-dependent, receiving SIMV of 4 with full cuff deflation and a Passy-Muir™ valve in-line with the ventilator tubing. He was maintained NPO when the assessment revealed a continued severe oropharyngeal dysphagia.

The patient now tolerated the speaking valve up to 3 hours a day and communicated functionally during these times.

Days 44 to 50

Weaning attempts progressed until the patient tolerated CPAP for all waking hours, and SIMV of 4 at night. He was placed on tracheostomy collar for 2-hour periods during the day. Joe wore the speaking valve consistently on and off the ventilator and was maintained with the cuff fully deflated. Oral communication was the primary method of communication. At night, when the patient was rested on the SIMV mode, the cuff was reinflated. He preferred to write and use

his word/phrase board to communicate at night. The tracheostomy tube was downsized to a No. 6 fenestrated tube with a fenestrated inner cannula. An oral diet was initiated after a reassessment of swallowing.

Days 50 to 55

Joe tolerated the use of a tracheostomy collar and a Passy-Muir™ valve during all waking hours by day 50. At night he was placed on CPAP with PSV. On day 54 the tube was capped for 2 hours during the day. He wore the speaking valve at other times to assist in the weaning process. Periods of capping were increased gradually. A tracheostomy collar was then used at night.

Days 55 to 60

Joe tolerated capping of the tracheostomy tube for all waking hours. He tolerated a soft diet and regular liquids. The tube was capped for 72 continuous hours, and he was successfully decannulated.

SUMMARY

Communication is an essential part of the treatment plan for the tracheostomized and ventilator-dependent patient. Often, communication goals can be met within the framework of other interests, such as weaning and decannulation. The speech-language pathologist plays an essential role on the team managing these challenging tasks.

REFERENCES

1. Santee JL. Psychosocial issues in the care of ventilator dependent patients: a patient's perspective. In: Mason M, ed. *Speech Pathology for the Tracheostomized and Ventilator-Dependent Patient.* Newport Beach, Calif: Voicing!; 1993: 424–432.

2. Kazandjian M, Dikeman K. Transdisciplinary team concept. In: Mason M, ed. *Speech Pathology for the Tracheostomized and Ventilator-Dependent Patient.* Newport Beach, Calif: Voicing!; 1993: 256–287.

3. Dikeman K, Kazandjian M. Managing tracheostomized and ventilator dependent adults: Current concepts. *ASHA Leader*, 2004;6–7:19–20.

4. Crimlisk JT, Wilson DJ. Artificial airways: a survey of cuff management practices. *Heart Lung.* 1996;25:225–235.

5. Bonanno PC. Swallowing dysfunction after tracheotomy. *Ann Surg.* 1971;174: 29–33.

6. Cameron JL, Reynolds J, Zuidema GD. Aspiration in patients with tracheostomies. *Surg Gynecol Obstet.* 1973;136: 68–70.

7. Feldman SA, Deal CW, Urquhart W. Disturbance of swallowing after tracheotomy. *Lancet.* 1966;1:954–955.

8. Siebens AA, Tippett DC, Kirby N, French J. Dysphagia and expiratory airflow. *Dysphagia.* 1993;8:266–269.

9. Tippett DC. More data needed to support cuff deflation. *Adv Speech-Lang Pathologists.* 1997;7(10):6.

10. Mason M, Meehan K. Tracheostomy and tracheostomy tubes. In: Mason M, ed. *Speech Pathology for the Tracheostomized and Ventilator-Dependent Patient.* Newport Beach, Calif: Voicing!; 1993: 126–183.

11. Eibling DE, Diez-Gross R. Subglottic air pressure: a key component of swallowing efficiency. *Ann Otol Rhinol Laryngol.* 1996;105:253–258.

12. Diez-Gross R, Mahlman J, Grayhack J. Physiologic effects of open and closed tracheostomy tubes on the pharyngeal swallow. *Ann Otol Rhinol Laryngol.* 2003;112(2):143–152.

13. Ikari T, Sasaki CT. Glottic closure reflex: control mechanisms. *Ann Otol Rhinol Laryngol.* 1980;89:220–224.

14. Buckwalter JA, Sasaki CT. Effect of tracheotomy on laryngeal function. *Otolaryngol Clin North Am.* 1984;17:41–48.

15. Colice GL. Resolution of laryngeal injury following translaryngeal intubation. *Am Rev Respir Dis*, 1992;145:361–364.

16. Barquist E, Brown M, Cohn S, Lundy, D, Jackowski J. Postextubation fiberoptic endoscopic evaluation of swallowing after prolonged endotracheal intubation: a randomized, prospective trial. *Crit Care Med.* 2001; 29,(9):1710–1713.

17. Heffner JE, Miller S, Sahn, SA. Tracheostomy in the intensive care unit: part 2. Complications. *Chest.* 1986; 90: 430–436.

18. Scalise P, Prunk S, Healy D, Votto J. The incidence of tracheoarterial fistula in patients with chronic tracheostomy tubes. *Chest.* 2005;128:3906–3909.

19. Dikeman KJ, Kazandjian MS. *Communication and Swallowing Management of Tracheostomized and Ventilator-Dependent Adults.* 2nd ed. Clifton Park, NY: Delmar-Thompson Learning; 2003: 185–190.

20. Siddharth P, Mazzarella L. Granuloma associated with fenestrated tracheostomy tubes. *Am J Surg.* 1985;150:279–280.

21. Snyderman CH, Johnson JT, Eibling DE. Laryngotracheal diversion and separation in the treatment of massive aspiration. *Curr Opin Otolaryngol Head Neck Surg.* 1994;2:63–67.

22. Dettelbach MA, Gross RD, Mahlmann J, Eibling DE. Effect of the Passy-Muir valve on aspiration in patients with tracheostomy. *Head Neck.* 1995;17(4):297–300.

23. Stachler RJ, Hamlet SL, Choi J, Fleming SM. *Scintigraphic quantification of aspiration with the Passy-Muir valve*. Paper presented at the Annual Convention of the American Academy of Otolaryngology Head and Neck Surgery; September 1994; San Diego, Calif.

24. Light RW, Aten JL, Fischer C, Chiang JT. Decannulation procedures for patients with chronic tracheostomies. *Chest*. 1989;96:257S.

25. Belozerco-Tracey L, Dikeman K, Harris, A, et al. *An interdisciplinary approach to tracheotomy capping and decannulation*. Presented at ASHA; November 2002; Atlanta, Ga.

26. Lichtman SW, Birnbaum IL, Sanfilippo MR, et al. Effect of a tracheostomy speaking valve on secretions, arterial oxygenation, and olfaction: a quantitative evaluation. *J Speech Hearing Res*. 1995;38:549–555.

27. Eliachar I. Unaided speech in long-term tube-free tracheostomy. *Laryngoscope*. 2000;110(5 pt1):749–760.

28. Bach JR. Alba A. Tracheostomy ventilation: a study of efficacy with deflated cuffs and cuffless tubes. *Chest*. 1990;97:679–683.

29. Tippett D, Siebens A. Speaking and swallowing on a ventilator. *Dysphagia*. 1991; 6:94–99.

30. Manzano JL, Lubillo S, Henriquez D, et al. Verbal communication of ventilator dependent patients. *Crit Care Med*. 1993;21:512–514.

31. Kazandjian MS, Dikeman KJ, Bach JR. Assessment and management of communication impairment in neurological disease. *Sem Neurol*. 1995;15:52–57.

32. Conway DH, Mackie C. The effects of tracheostomy cuff deflation during continuous positive airway pressure. *Anaesthesia*. 2004;59:652–657.

33. Goodenberger DM. Communication for the ventilator user with a tracheostomy. *Int Ventil Users Network*. 1993;7: 893–894.

34. Frey JA. *Weaning from mechanical ventilation augmented by the Passy-Muir speaking valve*. Paper presented at the American Lung Association/American Thoracic Society International Conference; May 1991; Anaheim, Calif.

35. Bell SD. Use of Passy-Muir tracheostomy speaking valve in mechanically ventilated neurological patients. *Crit Care Nurse*. 1996;16:63–68.

36. Nomori, H. Trachestomy tube enabling speech during mechanical ventilation. *Chest*. 2004;125(3):1046–1051.

37. Leder SB. Prognostic indicators for successful use of "talking" tracheostomy tubes. *Percept Motor Skills*. 1991;73: 441–442.

38. Drinker PA, Krupoff S. *Eyelink for nonvocal communication*. Paper presented at the Fourth Annual Conference on Rehabilitation Engineering; 1981; Washington, DC.

CHAPTER 12

Management of Swallowing Disorders in the Patient with a Tracheostomy

TAMARA WASSERMAN-WINCKO
RICARDO L. CARRAU

Any patient with a swallowing disorder should undergo an assessment that will provide information sufficient for the development of an individualized treatment plan. An ideal outcome is the return to an unrestricted oral diet; however, for many patients this starts with being able to participate in therapeutic feedings. Input from an experienced multidisciplinary team of specialists is critical to establish goals that are individualized for the patient's clinical situation and needs. Continual communication is necessary to refine these goals throughout the course of treatment according to the patent's needs and progress. An ideal team of specialists should include: primary care physicians, otolaryngologists, speech-language pathologists, nurses, respiratory therapists, nutritionists, and physical and occupational therapists.

The speech-language pathologist (SLP) begins the evaluation process by obtaining information from the medical chart and from discussions with nurses and physicians. In an alert and cooperative patient, a swallowing screening examination is completed to determine if instrumental testing, such as a modified barium swallow (MBS) and/or a fiberoptic endoscopic evaluation of swallowing (FEES) is necessary. Following the initial assessment, an individualized treatment plan is developed including the need for instrumental tests to obtain additional information.

A tracheostomy compounds the difficulty of the evaluation and treatment. Several reports have estimated that the frequency of aspiration in the patient with a tracheostomy ranges from 15 to 87%[1] and that silent aspiration may be present in 77% of patients who are mechanically ventilated.[2]

There are several theories as to why the swallowing function becomes compromised by a tracheostomy. Sasaki et al carried out tracheotomies in dogs and found that the laryngeal closure reflex is diminished when there is a loss of airflow through the larynx.[3] This suggests an impairment of the afferent-efferent reflex when an inflated cuff impedes the subglottic airflow and pressure. Without adequate efferent stimuli, the sphincteric mechanism of the glottis is insufficient and a cough response cannot be elicited to clear material that enters the airway or to prevent aspiration.

Laryngeal elevation, a term customarily used for the anterocephalic movement of the larynx produced by the contraction of the suprahyoid muscles, is one of the key components of a safe swallow. A tracheostomy may alter laryngeal elevation by its mechanical tethering effect and by causing pain. Inflated cuffs are thought to further anchor the larynx to the neck. In ventilator dependent patients, the ventilator tubing can weigh down on the tracheostomy tube, decreasing laryngeal elevation even more.[4,5] An overinflated cuff can compress the esophageal lumen, thus diverting food into the airway. Devita observed that swallowing problems may not necessarily be due to a mechanical problem, but rather due to muscle atrophy, weakness,

or poor muscle coordination.[6] In 2005, Ding and Logemann retrospectively studied a series of 623 patients with a tracheostomy and found that the frequency of silent aspiration and decreased laryngeal elevation was higher in patients with an inflated cuff.[7] Lastly, subglottic air pressure, present in normal subjects,[8] is disrupted by the presence of an open tracheostomy tube, and seems to contribute to aspiration risk also.

This chapter addresses what we consider to be the most important issues related to the assessment and management of the swallowing function in the patient with a tracheostomy. It covers the following topics: (1) preplanning, (2) noninstrumental testing, (3) instrumental testing, and (4) treatment options.

PREPLANNING

Preplanning is the first step in gathering information about the patient and using the knowledge accumulated from studies of patients who have had tracheostomy tubes. It also involves looking at the patient carefully and globally and consulting with the clinical care team. This provides guidance regarding when and how to proceed with the swallowing evaluation. Relevant questions that should be asked during this preliminary phase are: (1) What is the immediate goal? (2) What was the reason for the tracheostomy? (3) Is the tube cuffed and could the cuff be deflated? (4) Could the tube be downsized or removed? (5) Is the mechanical ventilation needed and if not, what is the expected duration of the weaning trials? (6) Is the patient a candidate for a speaking valve? (7) What is the prognosis for swallowing recovery? Answers to these questions will dictate how to proceed with the evaluation.

What Is the Immediate Goal?

Goals will vary based on the patient's general status, medical diagnoses, and prognosis for recovery. Patients in an acute care setting have problems, immediate needs, and goals that are very different from those seen in an outpatient clinic. ICU patients are medically compromised and in most cases need to be treated conservatively. Communication with the primary care team helps to establish the goals before proceeding with a full evaluation. The expectation may not be that the patient will return to an oral diet immediately, but to begin a rehabilitation program that will assist the patient in managing his or her own secretions, taking ice chips in moderation, and practice swallows to increase strength. Conversely, outpatients may be ready for an aggressive treatment plan that not only targets the mechanical issues related to the tracheostomy, but the underlying cause of the dysphagia.

What Is the Reason for the Tracheostomy?

Depending on the patient's medical condition, a tracheostomy may be temporary or permanent. The most common indication for a tracheostomy is prolonged ventilation or airway obstruction, which can either be acute or chronic. For example, some patients with cancer of the head and neck will have a tracheostomy tube placed at the time of surgery if the airway is compromised secondary to the effects of the cancer or to protect against postoperative edema. Once the edema subsides and the patient is able to manage his or her own secretions, the decannulation process begins. This usually implies a rapid change in the swallowing status and the possibility of starting therapy. Conversely, a patient with severe chronic obstructive pulmonary disease (COPD) or a quadriplegic patient may require a permanent or long-term tracheostomy as result of respiratory failure or the need for pulmonary toilet. Some of these patients will not tolerate weaning and will remain ventilator-dependent.

The goal is to assess the patient under optimal conditions. If a patient with cancer of the head and neck has difficulty swallowing after surgery, either secondary to edema or due to inability to manage his or her secretions, then it is prudent to defer the test for a few days. Patients who are ventilator-dependent, often benefit from going directly to instrumental testing.

Can the Cuff Be Deflated?

An inflated cuff prevents the exhaled air from entering the upper airway. Although a cuff may delay secretions from entering the lower airway, it does not prevent secretions from entering the larynx or the upper airway. Patients who are ventilator-dependent, however, usually require an inflated cuff. Nonventilator patients, or those weaning from the ventilator, may be candidates for cuff deflation if they do not require frequent suctioning.

The purpose of cuff deflation is to normalize airflow through the upper airway, restore laryngeal reflexes and cough, and to assess the patient's ability to use a one-way speaking valve for communication and swallowing. Once the cuff is deflated, the respiratory rate, oxygen saturation level, and patient's anxiety should be monitored to determine if the patient is ready to try a speaking valve.

What Is the Plan for Downsizing or Decannulation?

The adult tracheostomy tube size typically varies from 4.0- to 10.0-mm inner diameter and the outer diameter ranges from 9.4 to 14.0 mm. In general, patients with copious and/or thick secretions, require a larger tube for proper tracheal toilette. Once the secretions begin to diminish and the patient is able to tolerate a speaking valve for longer intervals, downsizing may be considered. Once the tracheostomy tube is downsized to a No. 4 cuffless tube, capping trials are initiated if the patient does not require the tracheostomy for any other reason. If the capping is tolerated for 24 hours without respiratory difficulty, then decannulation is done.

The presence of a tracheostomy tube and its size affect the patient's ability to swallow normally. As the larynx elevates and moves anteriorly, the upper esophageal sphincter opens to allow food/liquid to pass into the esophagus. If the larynx does not move adequately, the bolus may be retained in the pharynx placing the patient at risk for aspiration during or after the swallow. Downsizing may improve swallowing in several ways. A smaller tracheostomy tube may allow the patient to pass more air around the tube to the upper airway. This may help to restore the afferent-efferent reflexes

and may permit the use of a speaking valve more comfortably and to tolerate it for longer intervals during the day.

How Long Before the Patient Is Weaned from the Ventilator?

Careful attention should be given to the patient who is being weaned from mechanical ventilation. Patients who are beginning the weaning process and only tolerating it for short intervals, may not be good candidates for swallowing as the respiratory drive may override the coordination between breathing and swallowing. This increases the risk for aspiration, thus compromising the weaning and the patient's well being.

Swallowing should always be tested in conditions that are similar to those in which the patient is going to be eating. For example, if the patient is assessed while receiving mechanical ventilation and appears to do well, but receives food during a weaning trial, the change in circumstances may result in a change in function. The condition in which the patient is being assessed should always be documented in the chart.

Is the Patient Appropriate for a Speaking Valve Assessment?

Dettelbach et al suggested that a one-way speaking valve restores subglottic pressure and may improve swallowing.[9] In 1996, Stachler et al used scintigraphy to quantify the amount of aspirated material in 11 patients with a tracheostomy tube. The authors concluded that the amount of aspirated material, when the valve was on, was significantly less than when the tracheostomy was open.[10] Others have found that digital occlusion or the use of a speaking valve can decrease the risk of aspiration, although not in every patient. Logemann studied a series of 8 patients with cancer of the head and neck and tested the swallow with thin liquids and paste under videofluoroscopy with and without digital occlusion of the tracheostomy. She found 5 significant changes in swallow biomechanics by occluding the tracheostomy tube. These included: "(1) duration of base of tongue contact to the posterior pharyngeal wall was decreased, (2) maximal laryngeal elevation increased, (3) and (4) laryngeal and hyoid elevation at the time of the initial cricopharyngeal opening increased, and (5) onset of anterior movement of the posterior pharyngeal wall relative to the onset of cricopharyngeal opening occurred later."[11] Suiter et al tested 14 patients under videofluoroscopy under 3 conditions: (1) cuff inflated, (2) cuff deflated, and (3) one-way speaking valve. The 8-point penetration-aspiration scale was used to analyze each swallow. The results of her study described that there was a significant decrease in scores on the penetration-aspiration scale for thin liquid bolus with the speaking valve in place when compared to the cuff-inflated and cuff-deflated conditions.[12]

Patients who can use a speaking valve are at optimal condition for testing the swallow, but the evaluation should continue even if the valve cannot be worn. The valve allows the patient to produce an effective cough as long as the vocal folds are functioning properly. The cough is the protective mechanism of the larynx that clears the upper airway of aspiration if sensation is intact. Silent aspiration cannot be ruled out when the cuff is inflated; therefore, instrumental testing is necessary for proper assessment. Contraindications for the speaking valve include: foam cuff, severe tracheal/laryngeal stenosis, bilateral vocal fold paralysis, inability to tolerate cuff deflation, airway obstruction, unstable medical/pulmonary status, severe anxiety, and/or cognitive dysfunction.

What Is the Prognosis for Swallowing Recovery?

The prognosis for swallowing recovery depends on several factors. First, the medical diagnosis provides insight as to whether or not the swallowing problem will get progressively worse, if it is a temporary problem, or if the impairment will decline again at some point. For example, a patient admitted with exacerbation of a neurologic disorder, such as Parkinson's disease, will most likely require a longer course to recover swallowing function or may not be able to return to an oral diet of any kind due to the nature of the disease. Although a tracheostomy may be required to improve respiratory function, it often compounds the swallowing problem. The patient who has been nonoral for a lengthy period of time usually becomes deconditioned for swallowing and is at increased risk for aspiration. However, this type of swallowing impairment is usually temporary and should improve with time. These patients may include those with a gastrointestinal disease who must be nonoral until their medical condition improves, or those who have had a complicated medical course following a surgical procedure.

Another example of a temporary swallowing problem is when a vocal fold paralysis has been identified to be a significant contributor to the aspiration; once corrected with a vocal fold medialization, immediate improvement usually follows. The patient with cancer of the head and neck usually can obtain a functional level of swallowing following surgery; however, if the plan is to proceed with radiation therapy, a decline in swallowing function will occur if radiation is directed to specific areas that affect swallowing. Other factors to consider when determining prognosis are: the patient's cognitive status, positioning, and fatigue level during the assessment process. It is also important to note the patient's level of function during physical and occupational therapy (ie, ability to get out of bed, sit up in a chair, and walk). In addition, not all facilities have instrumental testing to determine if progress is being made, or have a team of specialists in the building that provide feedback about the patient's condition on a daily basis. In this situation, swallowing rehabilitation may proceed at a slower rate.

Estimating the prognosis is important because it will determine the need for temporary or long-term nutrition. Nutrition issues need to be addressed as early as possible to prevent delay in patient discharge. It is not unusual to monitor or reassess the patient before commenting on the prognosis of swallowing recovery, as patients conditions often change.

NONINSTRUMENTAL TESTING

Clinical Swallow Evaluation

The Clinical Swallow Evaluation (CSE) is the first step in the swallowing assessment process. It is usually considered a screening test because the information obtained from this examination is limited. For example, silent aspiration cannot be detected by the CSE.[13] The definition of silent aspiration is any material that enters the airway and falls below the vocal folds without a cough response. Furthermore, without being able to visualize the anatomic structures, one cannot rule out vocal fold paralysis, edema, or an obstruction that may interfere with the swallow process. The SLP cannot develop an optimal treatment plan without direct visualization of the physiology of the swallow. However, the following important information can be obtained: (1) the chief complaint; (2) current nutritional status; (3) appropriateness for ongoing assessment based on the case history and observation of the patient's participation and level of alertness; (4) if further testing is required, such as the modified barium swallow (MBS) or the fiberoptic endoscopic evaluation of swallowing (FEES); (5) if augmentative nutrition is required to meet caloric needs; and (6) if there is a need for modification or discontinuation of oral diet due to signs of dysphagia or aspiration.

Case History

A thorough case history is the first step in the swallowing evaluation. Information should be gathered from a patient interview, the medical chart, and the medical team. The examiner also needs to ascertain when the tracheostomy tube was placed, the type and size of tube, and the suctioning requirements. If the tube was recently inserted, it may be best to wait for at least 24 to 72 hours because patients often experience discomfort at the tracheostomy site.

Components of the Case History

Key components of the case history are presented in Tables 12–1 and 12–2.

First Step: Oral-Peripheral Exam

The oral-peripheral exam is the key component of a successful clinical swallowing evaluation. The goal is to assess the oral structures to determine whether there is a potential oral phase problem that would preclude using food and or drink as part of the evaluation. A cranial nerve examination is completed to evaluate sensory and motor function. During the examination, observations are made about oral hygiene, lingual and labial range of motion and strength, palatal elevation, and the management of oral secretions or the presence of xerostomia. If brief digital occlusion of the tracheostomy tube demonstrates that the patient is able to phonate, then observations can be made about vocal quality and ability to produce a cough. A breathy vocal quality and nonproductive cough can be signs of poor/reduced airway protection. If oral care is poor, such as crusting on the tongue/palate, or there is a presence of thick secretions, the swallowing assessment should be deferred until nursing care is provided. During the process of the oral-peripheral examination, the SLP can make note of patient participation, ability to follow instructions, respiration rate, speech intelligibility, and posture.

Second Step: Assessing the Swallow

Dikeman and Kazandijan highly recommend cuff deflation when assessing the

Table 12–1. Patient/Family Interview and Relevant Information from the Medical History

Chief complaint
Current Diet:
(a) oral vs nonoral
(b) type of diet
(c) type of augmentative nutrition
Onset and progression of dysphagia
Description of symptoms
Diet prior to hospitalization/dysphagia
History of pneumonia
History of weight loss
History of gastroesophageal reflux disease (GERD)
Hoarseness
Odynophagia
Results of previous swallowing studies or surgical intervention related to dysphagia

Table 12–2. Risk Factors Related to Dysphagia

History of radiation to head and neck due to cancer
Chronic obstructive pulmonary disease (COPD)
Neurologic disorders
Trauma
History of cervical spine surgery
Psychotropic and anticholinergic medications
Cervical osteophytes
Cognitive impairment

swallow.[14] If full cuff deflation is not possible, they recommend a partial cuff deflation. In some facilities, clearance from the attending physician is required before attempting any tracheostomy change. It is most prudent to discuss this with the primary medical team, whether it is a policy or not. Deep suctioning prior to cuff deflation and immediately following cuff deflation will remove secretions that may have been lying on top of the cuff. Deflating the cuff often restores sensation and should permit air to reach the true vocal folds, which can then elicit a cough, throat clearing, swallowing, and vocalization. If the patient is aphonic or presents with a breathy vocal quality and a weak cough, airway protection is most likely compromised, thus increasing the risk of aspiration. A consultation with an otolaryngologist is necessary to further evaluate laryngeal function before proceeding with swallowing trials of liquid or food. An SLP can make observations about laryngeal elevation and whether fatigue is a factor during saliva swallows. If the patient is able to demonstrate that he or she can manage secretions and is able to elicit a swallow, then the evaluation can progress to testing the swallow with ice chips and possibly other consistencies.

Third Step: Blue-Dye Testing

The tracheostomy tube can be useful for suctioning purposes and sometimes assists in the detection of aspiration. One method that might detect aspiration is the modified Evan's blue-dye test (MEBDT). The term blue-dye refers to FD&C Blue No. 1, or also known as "blue-food coloring." The MEBDT includes placing a few drops of blue dye on the patient's tongue to test for aspiration of secretions. Suctioning through the tracheostomy tube ensues on a regular basis and if the secretions are tinged blue, it may indicate a risk for pyrandial aspiration (refers to aspiration of food or liquid). Small amounts of blue-dye can also be placed in various consistencies, such as ice chips, liquids, or purees. It is recommended that this test should be done with one consistency at a time because a patient may show aspiration with one consistency and not another.[14] Several studies have shown that the blue-dye test has poor sensitivity and specificity. Thompson-Henry and Braddock reported false-negative results in 5 out 5 patients with a tracheostomy. The test did not identify aspiration that was later found on an instrumental swallow test.[15] Others have reported similar findings. Brady et al studied 20 tracheostomy patients with simultaneous MEBDT with MBS. Their results showed a 50% false-negative rate. The MEBDT identified aspiration in 100% of the patients who aspirated greater than 10% of the bolus, but did not detect aspiration of trace amounts.[16] Furthermore, Donzelli et al also found a 50% false-negative rate for detecting aspiration when comparing the MEBDT to the video nasal endoscopic examination. The MEBDT failed to reveal trace amounts of aspiration and only detected larger amounts that were aspirated in 67% of the patients.[17] Caution should be used with patients who have compromised pulmonary status when decisions are made based on blue-dye testing alone.

Blue-dye testing should only be used as a screening tool. Some clinicians do not have the luxury of specialized equipment that is used for swallowing evaluations and the blue-dye test, albeit its limitations, at least offers some insight.

Furthermore, the SLP cannot detect when and why aspiration occurred or the amount of residue in the pharynx that may lead to delayed aspiration. The lack of complete information obtained from this assessment limits the clinician's ability to develop a treatment plan that specifically focuses on the patient's problem.

Protocol for Blue Dye Testing— Adjunct to the Clinical Swallow Evaluation

The blue dye test is only a screening test and cannot rule out trace aspiration. The procedure may slightly vary from patient to patient based on their medical diagnosis and condition.

1. Proceed with oral examination and make observations about the patient (ie, ability to follow instructions, ability to participate in session, oxygen saturation level, and respiratory rate).
2. If the patient can tolerate cuff deflation, proceed with the speaking valve assessment. If the patient does not tolerate cuff deflation, reinflate the cuff and place a small amount of blue-dye on the patient's tongue to test for aspiration of secretions. Document the purpose for performing this task.
3. Once the speaking valve is placed, observe quality of voice and patient's ability to cough productively.
   - If the patient is aphonic or there is suspicion of vocal fold paralysis, request a fiberoptic endoscopic evaluation of swallowing (FEES).
   - Try dry test swallows and observe laryngeal elevation. If

the speaking valve is on, observe vocal quality and note if there are coughing episodes.
   - If the patient produces phonation and is comfortable with the valve in place, proceed with blue-stained ice-chips and continue with observations (bolus control, laryngeal elevation, swallows attempted per bolus, coughing during or after swallow attempts).
   - Suction
   - If negative, have nursing monitor for blue tracheal secretions for 24 hours (reason: residue can remain in the pharynx and can be aspirated later)
   - On Day 2, repeat the test and note if the patient's medical condition is the same. On day 2, other consistencies can be tried and same procedure is followed.
   - If there is any suspicion of aspiration, proceed to instrumental testing. (reason: trace aspiration is not always detected on the bedside evaluation)
   - A FEES or MBS should be done on all patients with a complicated medical history and who have not eaten orally for several weeks.

INSTRUMENTAL SWALLOWING EVALUATION

Fiberoptic Endoscopic Evaluation of Swallowing (FEES®)

FEES was first described in 1988 by Langmore[18] and the test is optimized when completed by an otolaryngologist and SLP following the clinical swallow evaluation. In some facilities the SLP can conduct the examination if the state licensure board permits it and if the clinician has received extensive training.

FEES involves placing an endoscope through the nasal cavity in order to directly visualize the pharynx and larynx before and after the swallow. The nose is decongested with oxymetazoline 0.05% and the anterior nose is anesthetized with viscous lidocaine applied with cotton applicators. Velopharyngeal closure is assessed prior to advancing the scope. Once the tip is in position above the epiglottis, observations are made regarding management of secretions, vocal fold mobility, airway protection, and possible signs of laryngopharyngeal reflux disease (LPRD). Abnormal findings such as a mass, granulomas, thrush, and anterior protrusion of the pharyngeal wall (often indicative of an anterior cervical osteophyte) can be detected during this examination. Swallowing function is assessed by using dyed boluses with the scope in place. The order and amount of food/liquid consistencies vary based on the diagnosis and condition of the patient. If the patient has penetration of material into the laryngeal vestibule and/or aspirates secretions, then food/liquid may be deferred. Patients are frequently asked to cough and to try to clear secretions within the laryngeal introitus so that airway clearance can be assessed directly.

Endoscopic observation can show the degree of posterior oral control, for example, food leaving the oral cavity before mastication. Pooling into the valleculae and or hypopharynx before the swallow occurs can indicate delayed initiation of the swallow or impaired pharyngeal response. Penetration into the laryngeal vestibule and aspiration before and/or after the swallow, postpharyngeal residue, and reflux from the esophagus back into the hypopharynx can be viewed directly (Fig 12–1). If any of these findings are observed, then swallowing maneuvers (ie, supraglottic swallow, super-supraglottic swallow, multiple swallows, effortful swallow, Mendelsohn) or postural techniques (chin tuck, head turns) are tried to decrease or eliminate residue and aspiration.

There are three primary limitations of this examination: (1) the oral phase is not directly observed, (2) the swallow itself cannot be viewed during the white-out phase, and (3) the UES and esophageal phase cannot be observed.

In summary, FEES is a useful tool that provides more information than the clinical swallow evaluation. It can be used multiple times without exposing the patient to radiation and is a good biofeedback tool during therapy. The test results can be stored and replayed for future comparisons. Therapeutic maneuvers and strategies can be implemented to improve

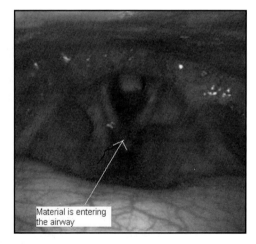

Fig 12–1. An FEES exam that demonstrates penetration in the supraglottic area and puree consistency beginning to enter the airway.

the efficiency of the swallow. The etiology of aspiration can be identified in most cases, which will allow the clinician to develop an individualized treatment plan focusing on specific goals. When in doubt if aspiration occurred, UES or lower dysfunction is suspected, or if swallowing biomechanics need to be observed directly, then a modified barium swallow or barium swallow should be completed.

Modified Barium Swallow Study (MBS)

The modified barium swallow (MBS), or videofluoroscopic study (VFS) was first described by Logemann in 1983.[19] The evaluation of swallowing function using ideofluoroscopy is also known as the "cookie swallow." However, this is misleading because a variety of other consistencies are now used. This examination is typically conducted by an SLP in conjunction with a radiologist or radiology technician. The MBS is considered to be the "gold standard" because it is a comprehensive evaluation of swallowing that views the oral, pharyngeal, and part of the esophageal phase of swallowing (Fig 12–2). The patient should be seated in their customary eating posture and viewed in the lateral and anterior position. The SLP usually administers various consistencies (thin liquids, thick liquids, pudding, and cookie) mixed with standardized amounts of barium. The order of consistencies and amount presented will depend on the patient's diagnosis and observed swallowing abilities.

Direct videofluoroscopic observation of swallowing permits the clinician to define oral and pharyngeal transit times, identify penetration and/or aspiration (before, during, and after the swallow), and the presence and location of oral and pharyngeal residue. Physiologic assessment is also possible, such as hyolaryngeal elevation, epiglottic inversion, retraction of the base of the tongue, and movement

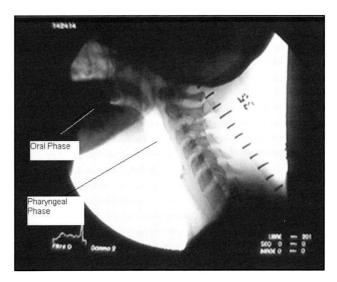

Fig 12–2. The lateral view of the MBS that primarily views the oral and pharyngeal phase of swallowing.

of the posterior pharyngeal wall. The MBS also determines whether or not osteophytes interfere with the swallow, if a Zenker's diverticulum is present, and if the upper esophageal sphincter (UES), is relaxing normally. Most importantly, the cause of aspiration and the risk factors can be identified immediately and strategies can be implemented during the examination to improve the efficiency and safety of the swallow.

TREATMENT OF DYSPHAGIA

Instrumental testing, such as the MBS and/or FEES, will provide the information needed to develop a treatment plan that will focus on specific goals related to the patient's oropharyngeal dysphagia. Once again, the input from the multidisciplinary team is very important during treatment planning for many reasons. First of all, some patients are only appropriate for therapeutic feedings with the SLP and will need augmentative nutrition to meet their needs. Others may be on a modified diet and may benefit from nutritional supplements. In either case, the dietician needs to be involved to address nutritional concerns. If the instrumental study indicates general deconditioning as a primary cause of the dysphagia, general strengthening programs provided by the physical therapists can be an effective adjunct to swallow treatment. The nursing staff needs to be aware of how the patient should be fed. If the patient shows improved swallow function with a speaking valve, benefits from specific feeding strategies or diet modifications, nursing needs to ensure that these recommendations are implemented for all meals.

Compensatory Intervention

During the instrumental evaluation, compensatory interventions are explored to determine their immediate effect on abnormal swallow findings. Compensatory strategies include*:

1. Posture change (chin tuck, head turn, head tilt). See Table 12–3.

---

*Refer to *Evaluation and Treatment of Swallowing Disorders*, Chapter 6 for a complete explanation of swallowing maneuvers.[19]

Table 12–3. Treatment Indication and Posture

Treatment Indications	Posture
Unilateral laryngeal/pharyngeal weakness or paralysis	Rotate head to the damaged side
Delayed pharyngeal swallow/reduced base of tongue	Chin tuck
Unilateral tongue damage	Head tilt to the stronger side
Poor or absent lingual propulsion	Tilt head back
Noncummulative residue in the pharynx	Lie on back or side

2. Swallow maneuvers (effortful swallow, supraglottic swallow, super-supraglottic swallow, Mendelsohn). See Tables 12–3, 12–4, and 12–5.
3. Increased sensory input (sour bolus, tactile stimulation, thermal stimulation). Indications for this

intervention is a swallow delay or diminished oral sensation
4. Modification of volume and speed of food presented. This intervention focuses on the size and the amount of the bolus, placement, and viscosity. Changing the food consistency is matching

Table 12–4. Treatment Indication and Swallow Maneuver

Treatment Indications	Maneuver
Weak base of tongue movement	Effortful swallow
Poor airway protection	Supraglottic swallow, super-supraglottic swallow
Poor hyolaryngeal elevation	Mendelsohn

Table 12–5. Description and Goal of Maneuvers

Maneuver	Explanation of Maneuver	Goal
Effortful swallow	Push tongue against the roof of the mouth and swallow hard. Squeeze muscles while swallowing.	To increase retraction of the base of tongue to posterior pharyngeal wall and to clear residue in the valleculae
Supraglottic swallow	1. Inhale and hold breath 2. Swallow while holding breath 3. cough	To increase airway protection by closing the true vocal folds before and during the swallow.
Super-supraglottic swallow	1. Inhale and hold breath tightly 2. Bear down 3. Swallow while holding breath and bearing down 4. Cough	To provide better airway protection by tilting the arytenoids to the epiglottis.
Mendelsohn	1. Begin to swallow 2. When you feel your Adam's apple rise, hold for several seconds 3. Follow through with the swallow	To increase the extent of laryngeal elevation which will increase relaxation of the UES.

the food to the physiology of the swallow.

5. Restoration of subglottic air pressure with digital occlusion, speaking valve, or capping of the tracheostomy tube.

Rehabilitative Intervention

Rehabilitative intervention focuses on improving the speed, force, or timing of structural movements. Therapy typically is completed over a 6- to 8-week period and then the patient is re-evaluated to determine if there is any change in swallowing function and if the goals have been met. If there has been surgical alteration of swallowing structures, then the patient may require prosthetic management to restore swallowing ability. See Table 12–6 for a listing of swallowing exercises and prosthetic management.

Table 12–6. Swallowing Exercises and Prosthetic Management

Identified Problem	Exercises	Explanation of Exercises	Prosthetic Appliance
Lingual weakness	Resistance (tongue blade or pressure bulbs)	Patient pushes tongue against the tongue blade/ bulbs for several seconds, relaxes, then repeats.	N/A
Reduced lingual-palatal contact	Lingual range of motion exercises	Patient is to move tongue in different directions to increase range of motion	Palatal drop (Figs 12–3 and 12–4)
>50% of tongue resected	Range of motion exercises for the residual tongue		Lingual prosthesis (Fig 12–5)
Reduced retraction of the base of tongue	Tongue hold maneuver	Patient places tongue between teeth and swallows	N/A
	Effortful swallow	See Table 12-3	
	Supraglottic swallow		
	Mendelsohn		
Incomplete vocal fold closure	Adduction exercises	Patient uses a hard glottal onset (ie, "go") and increase the loudness of the voice	N/A
	Lee Silverman program	Patient focuses on using a loud voice with sustained phonation	N/A

Table 12–6. *continued*

Identified Problem	Exercises	Explanation of Exercises	Prosthetic Appliance
Reduced hyolaryngeal elevation/ UES dysfunction	Falsetto-raises larynx	Patient slides up the pitch scale and holds for several seconds	N/A
	Mendelsohn (hyoid holding)	See Table 12–3	
	Shaker (head lifting exercise)	Patient lies flat on back, lifts neck, and looks at toes	
Velopharyngeal incompetence	Velar elevation exercises	Patient uses visual feedback and increased effort while lifting palate (eg, "ah") Patient uses an effortful /ka/ sound with words such as cake, cook, cup	Palatal lift (Fig 12–6)

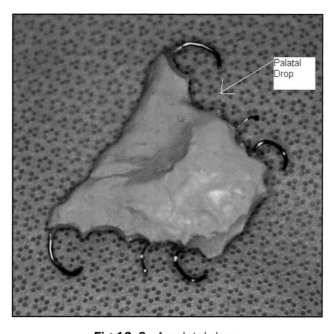

Fig 12–3. A palatal drop.

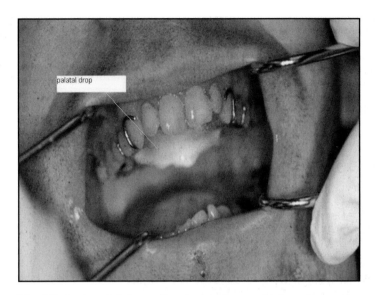

Fig 12–4. A palatal prosthesis in place, which reduces the volume in the oral cavity and allows better lingual–palatal contact for swallowing.

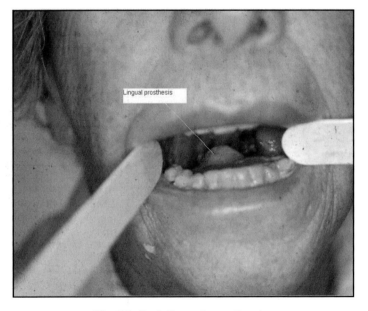

Fig 12–5. A lingual prosthesis.

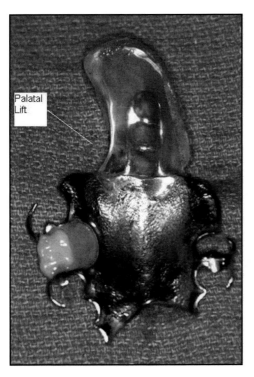

Fig 12–6. A palatal lift.

SURGICAL TREATMENT

Surgical treatment of swallowing disorders aims to improve velopharyngeal closure, glottic closure, UES opening, or to separate the airway from the foodway. Table 12–7 summarizes surgical procedures for dysphagia.

SUMMARY

When a tracheostomy tube is present, the steps in conducting the evaluation become more complex than the basic swallow evaluation. An understanding of the effects of the presence of a tracheostomy tube on swallowing function is necessary to proceed with the evaluation appropriately. Management of swallowing

Table 12–7. Surgical Procedures for Dysphagia

Identified Problem	Procedure	Purpose
Velopharyngeal incompetence (VPI)	Palatopexy Palatal adhesion Palatal flap	To improve velopalatine closure.
Vocal fold paralysis, atrophy, or paresis	Vocal fold injection Laryngeal framework surgery	To improve glottic closure.
Incomplete UES opening	Botox Dilatation Cricopharyngeal myotomy	To facilitate the passage of the bolus into the esophagus.
Recurrent aspiration pneumonia	Laryngotracheal separation	Separates respiratory from alimentary tract

disorders in the patient with a tracheostomy can be accomplished with a multidisciplinary team approach. The speech-language pathologist has the primary responsibility of assessing the swallow and determining the most appropriate treatment plan that will help the patient achieve his or her goals.

REFERENCES

1. Elpern EH, Jacobs ER, Bone RC. Incidence of aspiration in tracheally intubated adults. *Heart Lung.* 1987;16(5):527-531.

2. Elpern EH, Scott MG, Petro L, Ries MH. Pulmonary aspiration in mechanically ventilated patients with tracheostomies. *Chest.* 1994;105(2):563-566.

3. Sasaki CT, Suzuki M, Horiuchi M, Kirchner JA. The effect of tracheostomy on the laryngeal closure reflex. *Laryngoscope.* 1977;87(9 pt 1)1428-1433.

4. Bonanno PC. Swallowing dysfunction after tracheostomy. *Ann Surg,* 1971; 174(1):29-33.

5. Feldman SA, Deal CW, Urquhart W. Disturbance of swallowing after tracheostomy. *Lancet.* 1966;1(7444):954-955.

6. DeVita MA, Spierer-Rundback L. Swallowing disorders in patients with prolonged orotracheal intubation or tracheostomy tubes. *Crit Care Med.* 1990;18(12): 1328-1330.

7. Ding R, Logemann JA. Swallow physiology in patients with trach cuff inflated or deflated: a retrospective study. *Head Neck.* 2005;27(9):809-813.

8. Gross RD, et al. Direct measurement of subglottic air pressure while swallowing. *Laryngoscope.* 2006;116(5):753-761.

9. Dettelbach MA, Gross RD, Mahlman G, Eibling DE. Effect of the Passy-Muir valve on aspiration in patients with tracheostomy. *Head Neck.* 1995;17(4): 297-302.

10. Stachler RJ, et al. Scintigraphic quantification of aspiration reduction with the Passy-Muir valve. *Laryngoscope.* 1996; 106(2 Pt 1):231-234.

11. Logemann JA, Pauloski BR, Colangelo L. Light digital occlusion of the tracheostomy tube: a pilot study of effects on aspiration and biomechanics of the swallow. *Head Neck.* 1998;20(1):52-57.

12. Suiter DM, McCullough GH, Powell PW. Effects of cuff deflation and one-way tracheostomy speaking valve placement on swallow physiology. *Dysphagia.* 2003; 18(4):284-292.

13. Peruzzi WT, et al. Assessment of aspiration in patients with tracheostomies: comparison of the bedside colored dye assessment with videofluoroscopic examination. *Respir Care.* 2001;46(3):243-247.

14. Dikeman KJ, Kazandjian MS. *Comunication and Swallowing Management of Tracheostomized and Ventilator-Dependent Adults.* 2nd ed. Clifton Park, NY: Thompson Delmar Learning; 2003:292, 294

15. Thompson-Henry S. Braddock B. The modified Evan's blue dye procedure fails to detect aspiration in the tracheostomized patient: five case reports. *Dysphagia.* 1995;10(3):172-174.

16. Brady SL, Hildner CD, Hutchins BF. Simultaneous videofluoroscopic swallow study and modified Evans blue dye procedure: an evaluation of blue dye visualization in cases of known aspiration. *Dysphagia.* 1999;14(3):146-149.

17. Donzelli J, Brady S, Wesling M, Craney M. Simultaneous modified Evans blue dye procedure and video nasal endoscopic evaluation of the swallow. *Laryngoscope.* 2001;111(10):1746-1750.

18. Langmore SE, Skarupski KA, Park PS, Fries BE. Predictors of aspiration pneumonia in nursing home residents. *Dysphagia.* 2002;17(4):298-307.

19. Logemann J. *Evaluation and Treatment of Swallowing Disorders.* Austin, Tex: Pro-Ed. 1986;198-201, 214-221.

Index